I Remember...

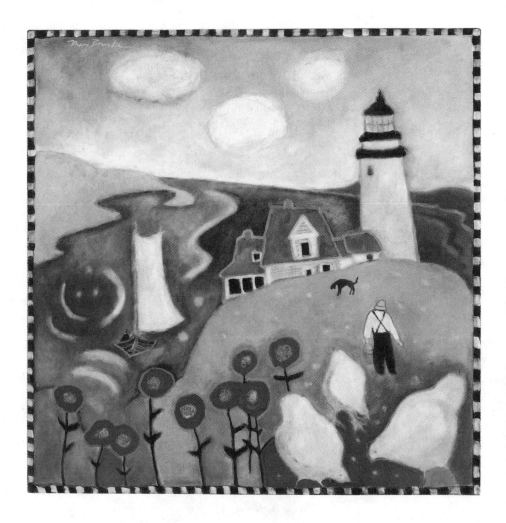

Recipes & Memories

Collected by
The Maine Alzheimer's Association

By The Maine Alzheimer's Association

For information about obtaining additional
copies of *I Remember*...contact

The Maine Alzheimer's Association
163 Lancaster Street, Suite 160B
Portland, Maine 04101-2406

Night or day, one phone call away...
Call our 24/7 Helpline at 1-800-660-2871.

First Printing   October 1999
Second Printing   December 2000
Third Printing   April 2002
Fourth Printing   June 2003
Fifth Printing   April 2006

ISBN 0-9674712-0-6

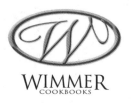

WIMMER
COOKBOOKS

ConsolidatedGraphics
1-800-548-2537

Introduction

"I Remember . . ." was born at a festive baby shower luncheon with the staff and volunteers of the Maine Alzheimer's Association. The room was filled with shower gifts as well as delicious potluck dishes that everyone brought to share. Someone said, "This meal is wonderful—we ought to write a cookbook!" And the rest, as they say, is history.

"I Remember . . ." is a celebration of the special people and special moments in our lives. We built the book on the theme of memories—memories of gatherings with great food, family and friends. This theme touched a chord for hundreds of people who became involved in the process.

What started as a little project over lunch became a tremendous undertaking that brought together a large steering committee as well as recipe contributors, testers, typists, proofreaders, artists and graphic designers. A Maine artist, whose painting evoked for us the theme of memories and home, allowed us to use her work on our cover. There is something about the Maine Alzheimer's Association that brings out the best in people; we are humbled by the tremendous outpouring of support for this project and grateful to all those who participated.

The response to our request for recipes was overwhelming. We were warned by our publisher that soliciting recipes would be the most difficult task and to expect no more than 200. We received over 500 recipes in a three-month period, which came from 88 cities and towns in Maine as well as 18 states. Recipes were tested, and since this is a community effort, we made the decision to include at least one recipe from every contributor. The range of recipes includes simple, quick and easy meals as well as comfort foods and entrées for special dinner parties. There is a special emphasis on Maine recipes that takes advantage of our abundant native resources and local specialties.

In the end, this project captured the hearts of many that have experienced the effects of Alzheimer's disease within their families, among their friends, in their communities. As one of our committee members stated so beautifully, "This dreadful disease may claim the memory of a loved one, but it holds no power over our memories of them." Memories are very important at the Maine Alzheimer's Association, but so is our hope for the future. We think you will delight in our recipes and stories for many years to come.

The Organization

The Maine Alzheimer's Association is dedicated to supporting people with Alzheimer's disease and their caregivers by fostering a greater understanding of the disease through a variety of programs, services and advocacy efforts.

We stand by the people of Maine to assist them through the journey of Alzheimer's. Our programs and services include a toll-free Helpline as well as education and training of families, professionals, clergy, and law enforcement personnel. We offer a Family Connections Program, over 40 support groups throughout the state and numerous community outreach programs. Our voices are heard in the state legislature and in Congress when issues affecting people with Alzheimer's and their families arise, and we are committed to supporting research that will reduce the impact of Alzheimer's disease and eventually eliminate it.

The most common form of dementia, Alzheimer's disease is a progressive, degenerative disease in which brain cells die and are not replaced. It results in impaired memory, thinking and behavior, affecting a person's personality, the ability to perform routine activities and to live independently. Approximately 4 million Americans have Alzheimer's disease. It is the fourth leading cause of death for adults in the U.S. Though it can affect people in their 40's and 50's, the risk of developing the disease increases with age. An estimated 14 million people will have Alzheimer's disease by the year 2050 if no prevention or treatment is found. In Maine, Alzheimer's disease or a related dementia affects approximately 30,000 people.

The Alzheimer's Association has a vision: to create a world without Alzheimer's disease while optimizing the quality of life for individuals and their families. Our mission is to provide leadership to eliminate Alzheimer's through the advancement of research, while enhancing care and support services for individuals and their families. To that end, the Maine Alzheimer's Association serves as a resource to persons with Alzheimer's disease, their families and caregivers.

A small but dedicated staff and a greater number of volunteers, many of whom have been touched by the disease, carry out the work of the Maine Alzheimer's Association. Volunteers serve as Board and committee members, answer the Helpline, provide office and computer support, participate in our events, raise money, testify in legislative hearings and more. This cookbook represents another herculean effort by many wonderful volunteers that the Maine Alzheimer's Association is blessed to include in its family.

The Alzheimer's Association is a non-profit, tax-exempt organization founded in 1980. It is the only national voluntary health organization dedicated to research, and to providing support and assistance to people with Alzheimer's disease, their families and caregivers.

Cookbook Committee

Members of this committee created this book. They attended planning meetings, served as recipe solicitors, recipe testers, design consultants, typists, editors and proofreaders.

Kathleen Leslie and Susan Braziel, *Co-Chairs*

Susan Arnold	Ann Noyes
Vera Berv	Gail Pelletier
Dot Cleveland	Janet Richardson
Sarah deDoes	Sally Sewall
Hillary Dorsk	Joan Stockford
Eleanor Goldberg	Liz Weaver
Susan Grondin	Tish Whipple
Carolyn McGoldrick	Margaret Wilkis
Tonia Medd	

Additional Recipe Testers

Jacquie Black	Krista Martin
Judy Calise	Claudia Monsell
Joan Dinsmore	Karen O'Brien
Dorette Frank	Linda Painchaud
Linda Green	Sally Subilia
Chris Gunderman	Cassandra Wright
Susan Leslie	

Additional Typists and Proofreaders

Marjorie Jamback
typist

Melody MacDonald
proofreader

Special Thanks

Mary Bourke
Artist

Jill Eaton
Small Pond Studios

Peggy Golden
Greenhut Galleries

Mary Taddia
Maine Alzheimer's Association

Jay York
Affordable Photo

About the Cover Artist

Mary Bourke has been painting all her life, since she was a little girl growing up in a family of 9 children in Port Washington, New York. Her older brother was an artist who took her along to his art lessons. She attended school in Boston, moved north after graduation, back to New York in the '80s, and now resides in Lincolnville, Maine, where she has been an art teacher, but now paints full time. Her latest work depicts simple, nostalgic themes of family and home which revolve around snapshots from the '50s of her own childhood home. She often incorporates into her paintings something from the long-ago past, like the "square sail" in the painting on the cover of this book.

Table of Contents

Try

Tomato Tart — p. 65
Lg. breakfast casseroles — pgs. 68-9
Parsnip Soup — p. 92
Carrot sandwich spread — p. 111
Bugullion (Shirley (Orbe)) — p. 166 — for kids
Garlic Roasted Lamb — p. 167
Lamb Shanks a la Greque — p. 170
chicken recipes — 172-3, 179, most of them, 184
Turkey breast — 191; Cornish Game Hens — 192
Salmon Loaf — 200
Scrod — 214
Eggplant / Tomato Au Gratin — 247

Appetizers

Cheese with Pungent Cherry Chutney Sauce

Preparation Time: 15 minutes

10 or more appetizer servings

1	cup dried cherries
1	cup brown sugar
¾	cup balsamic vinegar
2	tablespoon orange juice concentrate
	Brie or cream cheese
	Toasted slivered almonds
	Crackers

Combine cherries, balsamic vinegar and brown sugar in sauce pan. Simmer for 10 to 15 minutes. Add orange juice. Return to heat and simmer 5 minutes. Remove from burner. Cool slightly before pouring over Brie or formed cream cheese. Sprinkle with slivered almonds. Serve with crackers.

Tish Whipple
Portland, Maine

Note: Sauce can also be used as a wonderful glaze for a chicken or pork dish.

Homemade Boursin

"A favorite recipe for family get-togethers or to take on boat cruises."

Preparation Time: 10 minutes

1½ pounds

1   8-ounce container whipped butter, softened
2   8-ounce packages cream cheese, softened
½   teaspoon garlic powder
¼   teaspoon marjoram leaves
¼   teaspoon basil
¼   teaspoon celery seed
¼   teaspoon dill seed
¼   teaspoon oregano
¼   teaspoon seasoned salt
    Dry Sherry
    Crackers or sturdy chips

Mix all ingredients well. Splash some dry sherry in to help mix smoothly. (Do not use beater, mixer or food processor for this recipe.) Shape into a ball. Wrap and store in refrigerator. It will keep several weeks covered. Bring to room temperature before serving. Serve with crackers or chips.

Joanne Bingham
Scarborough, Maine

Holiday Cheese Ball

"This is a family tradition during the holidays. I always use 2 tablespoons Tabasco because it gives it a great 'kick'! We all like it with a lot of Tabasco, even my Dad who always notices the 'bite.'"

Preparation Time: 20 minutes plus refrigeration

1 large or 2 small balls

2	8-ounce packages cream cheese, softened
1	cup shredded cheddar cheese
1	cup shredded ham
1	green pepper, finely diced
1	small onion, finely diced
2	teaspoons to 2 tablespoons Tabasco
2	tablespoons dried parsley flakes
1	cup ground walnuts
	Crackers

In large bowl mix cream cheese, cheddar cheese, ham, green pepper and onion. (It is easier if you use your hands.) Add parsley flakes and Tabasco. Form into ball(s), roll in ground walnuts, wrap in plastic wrap and refrigerate until set (a couple of hours). Serve with crackers.

Cheri Alexander
Boothbay, Maine

Tester's Note: Delicious flavor. Gets even better with time. Suggest making it at least a day ahead.

curry Cheese and chutney spread

"Given to me by a friend in the Old Greenwich Newcomers Club 20 years ago. It has become a family favorite."

Preparation Time: 30 minutes

10 to 12 servings

1	6-ounce package cream cheese, softened
1	cup sharp cheddar cheese, shredded
4	teaspoons dry sherry
¼	teaspoon curry powder
1	tablespoon chopped onion
½	cup plum (or other) jam
¼	cup golden raisins
1	tablespoon red wine vinegar
½	teaspoon pumpkin pie spice
	Wheat crackers

Mix the first five ingredients well until smooth. Shape into a volcano on your serving plate. Cook the jam, raisins, vinegar and spice until mixed well. Cool. Pour over cheese mix and serve with wheat crackers.

Joanne O. Bingham
Scarborough, Maine

Vidalia Onion Spread

"A favorite recipe in Georgia when those Vidalias come in."

Preparation Time: 10 minutes

Baking Time: 15 to 20 minutes

3 cups

1   cup chopped onion (Vidalia preferred)
1   cup shredded Swiss cheese
1   cup mayonnaise
    Crackers

Preheat oven to 325°. Mix ingredients and bake 15 to 20 minutes, until firm. Serve hot with crackers.

Susan Arnold
Portland, Maine

Walnut Pâté

"Perfect recipe for the vegetarian"

Preparation Time: 35 minutes

8 to 10 servings

2   onions
3   eggs
1   cup walnuts
1   can tiny early peas
1   tablespoon oil
1   teaspoon garlic powder
    Salt and pepper to taste

Chop onions. Sauté in oil. Hard boil eggs. Grind walnuts very fine. Drain peas. Put all ingredients in food processor, add seasonings and process to pâté texture (can use hand blender).

Irma Goldberg
Chicago, Illinois

Pâté Maison

"A French tradition and one of my husband's favorite holiday recipes. His mother first taught me how to make it."

Preparation Time: 1½ to 2 hours

10 or more appetizer servings

1 medium onion
1 clove garlic, cut in half
1 cup milk
1 pound ground pork
1 cup coarse bread crumbs (2 slices day-old bread)
1 teaspoon seasoned salt
½ teaspoon pepper
½ teaspoon celery salt
⅛ teaspoon cinnamon
⅛ teaspoon sugar
  Dash of sage
  Crackers

Process onion, garlic and milk in blender until smooth. Combine with remaining ingredients in a heavy Dutch oven. Mix well. Cover and simmer on very low heat for an hour, stirring frequently and breaking up chunks. Cool slightly. Pour half the mixture into a blender and process a few seconds until smooth. Repeat with remaining mixture. Pour into a very lightly oiled 3-cup mold. Cover and chill until firm. Unmold by inverting on a serving platter. Serve with crackers.

Shirley Bastien
Skowhegan, Maine

Tester's Note: Excellent. Preferring the pâté less smooth, we omitted the last step of mixing in the blender.

Seafood Pizza Dip

Preparation Time: 15 to 20 minutes

2 dozen appetizer servings

½ cup mayonnaise
1   8-ounce package cream cheese
½ cup sour cream
1   cup seafood cocktail sauce
1   6-ounce can tiny shrimp, rinsed and drained
1   large tomato, seeds removed and finely chopped
1   large green pepper, finely chopped
1   cup shredded mozzarella cheese
    Crackers

Beat the first three ingredients together well. Spread in large round non-metal tray. Top with seafood cocktail sauce. Spread shrimp over sauce. Sprinkle tomato and green pepper over shrimp. Add mozzarella cheese over pepper and tomato. Seal with plastic wrap and refrigerate. Best done ahead of time. Serve with your favorite crackers.

Stella Ouellette
Frenchville, Maine

**Note: This recipe works well with all low fat ingredients.
May use 2 smaller dishes instead of one large dish.**

Spicy Corn Dip

"My friend and former co-worker, Dan, was diagnosed with Alzheimer's several years ago. He was once a gifted writer and storyteller who loved a good joke and was the life of the party. One time I had to make a quick appetizer for a party in our department so I threw together a batch of 'Sauced Dogs'. These were cocktail wieners in a sauce made of, among other things, a healthy shot of Jack Daniels. After his retirement, he called me at work about 10:30 one morning and said, 'Hey, can you give me your recipe for Sauced Dogs?' I said, 'Sure, what are you making them for?' After a deliberate pause, he replied, 'Lunch!' My tastes have changed somewhat and now my contribution to party fare is much more likely to be either a hot crab dish or this wonderful Spicy Corn Dip. But when I flip through my recipes, I stop at the Sauced Dogs and remember Dan and long for him to still be the life of the party."

Preparation Time: 30 minutes

3 dozen appetizer servings

1   16-ounce bag frozen white corn
1   8-ounce package cream cheese, softened
½   cup sour cream
2   tablespoons cumin
1   cup Monterey Jack cheese, shredded
½   cup finely chopped red pepper
2   tablespoons chopped pickled jalapeño pepper
2   tablespoons chopped cilantro
    Salt and pepper to taste
    Tortilla chips

Cook corn approximately five minutes; drain. Combine corn with softened cream cheese, sour cream and cumin, stirring until blended. Fold in shredded cheese, peppers and cilantro. Salt and pepper to taste. Serve at room temperature with tortilla chips.

Ardith Bradshaw, Publishing Consultant
Memphis, Tennessee

California Taco Dip

Preparation Time: 30 minutes

Enough for 20 people

1	15-ounce can refried beans
1	package taco seasoning mix
2	tablespoons salsa
1	8-ounce container plain yogurt
2	small avocados, mashed
1	squeeze of lemon juice
1	4-ounce can diced peeled green chilies
1	tomato, diced
1	bunch spring onions, chopped
1½	cups shredded Monterey Jack cheese
20-30	black olives, sliced
	Tortilla chips

Prepare by layering ingredients in a deep dish pie plate.

1st layer: Refried beans, taco seasoning, salsa

2nd layer: Yogurt, avocados, lemon juice

3rd layer: Green chilies, tomatoes, spring onions

4th layer: Shredded cheese and black olives

Refrigerate until ready to use. Serve with tortilla chips.

Joe Sirois
Rumford, Maine

Baked Taco Dip

"The Subilia Family is famous among friends for their campfires. Parents and children join in to share an evening of friendship and family fun. People bring an appetizer or dessert to complete the meal. This tasty dip was contributed by a good friend, Julie Stevens."

Preparation Time: 10 minutes

Baking Time: 20 minutes at 350°

8 to 10 servings

1   8-ounce package cream cheese, softened
1   15-ounce can low fat refried beans
1   8-ounce package taco cheese
    Shredded lettuce, tomatoes, diced olives as toppings
      (optional)
    Nacho chips

Preheat oven to 350°. Spread cream cheese in bottom of greased pie plate. Add refried beans and spread over cream cheese. Top with taco cheese. Bake for approximately 20 minutes. Serve hot with nacho chips.

Sally Subilia
Wells, Maine

Note: Sharp cheddar cheese may be used if taco cheese is too hot. It is also an option to mix chopped zucchini or summer squash, raw or roasted, into the cream cheese before spreading.

Mexican Cheese Dip

Preparation Time: 20 minutes

30 servings

1   2-pound block of processed cheese loaf
1   pound breakfast sausage (Jimmy Dean Hot works best)
1   14½-ounce can Mexican-style tomatoes, chopped
    Tortilla chips
    Sliced jalapeño peppers (optional)

Fry sausage until no longer pink. Drain fat well. Microwave cheese and tomatoes until melted. Add sausage and mix thoroughly. Serve with tortilla chips. Throw in sliced jalapeños for an extra "zing".

Rose Buse Ross
Rumford, Maine

Hot Cheese and Onion Dip

Preparation Time: 10 minutes

Baking Time: 20 minutes

1   8-ounce stick cheddar cheese grated
1   cup Hellmann's mayonnaise
1   small onion, grated
    Crackers or vegetables

Preheat oven to 400°. Mix all ingredients together. Put into a small, greased casserole dish, and bake for 20 minutes or until bubbly and golden. Serve with crackers or raw vegetables.

Janet Philbrick
Cape Elizabeth, Maine

Note: This recipe freezes well.

Baked Pepperoni Pizza Dip

"Kids love this. Better make two!"

Preparation Time: 30 minutes

Baking Time: 15 to 20 minutes

8 to 10 appetizer servings

1 8-ounce package cream cheese, softened
1¼ cups shredded mozzarella cheese, divided
½ cup sour cream
1 teaspoon oregano
⅛ teaspoon garlic powder
½ cup pizza sauce
½ cup chopped pepperoni
¼ cup sliced green onion
¼ cup chopped green pepper

Mix cream cheese, ¾ cup mozzarella, sour cream, oregano and garlic powder; spread on bottom of pie or quiche plate. Spread pizza sauce on this mix. Sprinkle pepperoni, onion and green pepper on top. Bake 10 to 15 minutes. Top with remaining mozzarella cheese and bake 5 minutes more.

Barb Viti
Augusta, Maine

Hot Crabmeat Dip

"My son has requested this for his birthday dinner appetizer for more years than any of us can remember."

Preparation Time: 10 minutes

Baking Time: 30 minutes

6 to 8 servings

2   8-ounce packages cream cheese, softened
6   ounces crabmeat
1   teaspoon half-and-half
    Salt and white pepper
    Crackers or raw veggies

Preheat oven to 350°. Mix half-and-half into softened cream cheese. Mix in crabmeat. Mix in salt and white pepper to taste. Spread into 8 or 9-inch pan. The mixture should be ½ to 1-inch thick. Serve with crackers or raw veggies.

Sarah deDoes
Portland, Maine

Crab Fondue

Preparation Time: 15 minutes

8 to 10 appetizer servings

½   stick butter
1   8-ounce block processed cheese loaf
6   ounces fresh crabmeat
    Hot sauce to taste (optional)
    Crackers

Melt butter over medium heat with cheese. Add fresh crabmeat. Stir well. Transfer to fondue dish. Keep warm. Serve with your favorite crackers.

Eileen Flanagan
Rockland, Maine

Crab Imperial

Preparation Time: 20 minutes

Broiling Time: 3 to 5 minutes

8 servings

1	small onion, chopped
¼	cup butter
2	tablespoons flour
½	cup milk
½	cup half-and-half
⅛	teaspoon red pepper
⅛	teaspoon nutmeg
2	tablespoons dry sherry
¼	cup mayonnaise
2	teaspoons lemon juice
1	pound crabmeat
	Parmesan cheese
	Paprika

Preheat broiler. Sauté onion in butter for 5 minutes. Add flour and whisk with butter and onion. Stir in milk, half-and-half, seasonings and sherry. Cook on medium heat until thickened and smooth. Remove from heat and add mayonnaise and lemon juice. Stir in crabmeat. Spoon into shells that have been slightly buttered. Top with Parmesan cheese and paprika. Brown under broiler 3 to 5 minutes.

L'Ermitage
Bucksport, Maine

Marinated Shrimp

"My grown children still expect this dish at special occasions - Thanksgiving, Christmas, birthdays, etc."

Preparation Time: 15 to 20 minutes

24 appetizer servings

6	pounds cooked and peeled shrimp
3	pounds onions, sliced
2	cups salad oil
	Juice of 18 lemons
1½	cups catsup
½	cup chopped parsley
1	cup granulated sugar
3	cloves garlic, minced (optional)
4	lemons or oranges, sliced
¼-½	teaspoon dry mustard
	Salt and pepper

Combine all ingredients. Marinate in refrigerator one week. Good as a first course or as an hors d'oeuvre. Best made at least two days ahead.

Elaine Fantle Shimberg
Scarborough, Maine

Tester's Note: The sweet and sour taste is a tangy treat! Color is bright with pink shrimp, red sauce and flecks of green parsley. If you buy fresh uncooked shrimp, add 15 minutes to the prep time for peeling and 6 to 8 minutes for broiling.

Seared Maine Diver Scallop with Golden Raisins and Chervil

Preparation Time: 10 minutes

4 servings

4	large Maine diver scallops
1	cup of Chenin Blanc white wine
½	cup golden raisins
4	tablespoons unsalted butter
2	tablespoons fresh chervil
	Sea salt and ground black pepper to taste
	Polenta and field greens (optional)

Soak raisins in wine until plump (about one hour). Season scallops with salt and pepper. Get a sauté pan very hot and place a small amount of oil in the bottom. Quickly sear scallops in pan until golden brown (about a minute on each side) and remove from pan. Add raisin wine mixture and butter to pan; reduce for a minute. Place scallops back into pan with chervil for a second to heat back up. Place each scallop on a serving plate and spoon the sauce over top. May garnish each plate with a little polenta and/or field greens, if desired.

Gabriel's (Gabriel Bremer)
Portland, Maine

Coquilles Nantaise

"This is an original recipe of L'Ermitage."

Preparation Time: 20 minutes

Baking Time: 10 to 12 minutes

8 servings

2 pounds scallops
6 shallots, minced
1 stick butter, melted
1 tablespoon parsley
½ cup bread crumbs

Preheat oven to 400°. Wash scallops; remove vein. Slice into small pieces. Sauté shallots until soft in 2 tablespoons butter. Add remaining ingredients. Put ¼ cup filling into each of 8 buttered clam shells. Bake for 10 to 12 minutes.

L'Ermitage
Bucksport, Maine

Water Chestnuts Wrapped in Bacon

"These are fun to make. We used to have a lot of laughs making these. While people were in the living room socializing, we'd be in the kitchen eating them as fast as we were making them!"

Preparation Time: 10 minutes

8 to 10 servings

2 8-ounce cans whole water chestnuts
½-1 pound bacon
1-1½ cups Teriyaki sauce

Wrap ½ to 1 slice bacon around each water chestnut. Secure with toothpick and dip all sides in Teriyaki sauce, then microwave 2 to 2½ minutes.

Anita Reardon
Gray, Maine

Pita Snack

Preparation Time: 10 minutes

Baking Time: 20 minutes

1   package 7-inch pita breads (wheat or white)
1   stick butter or margarine, softened
     Garlic salt to taste

Preheat oven to 325°. Split each pita bread into 2 pieces (will have 8 round pieces). Spread each piece with softened butter or margarine. Sprinkle each piece with garlic salt. Bake for 15 to 20 minutes. When cooking, check for signs of browning. Cut pieces into bite size pieces with scissors. Cool. Can be stored in plastic bags. Will keep a week or more. When ready to use, warm in slow oven 200° for 30 minutes.

Barbara Pratt
Scarborough, Maine

Tester's Note: You can substitute real minced garlic (2 cloves) plus 1 teaspoon salt for the garlic salt.

Swiss Cheese and Walnut Strudel

"I love appetizers and this is one of the best. Leftovers make a great lunch the next day."

Preparation Time: 1 hour

Baking Time: 30 minutes

8 to 10 servings

Pastry
1¾ cups flour
1   teaspoon salt
2   tablespoons sugar
10 tablespoons butter or margarine
2   tablespoons shortening
⅓   cup cold water

Cheese Nut Filling
1½ cups grated Swiss cheese
½   cup chopped walnuts
1   egg
1   tablespoon Worcestershire sauce
1   teaspoon fresh minced garlic
½   teaspoon onion powder
¼   teaspoon each oregano, thyme, and basil
½   teaspoon dry mustard

Egg Glaze
1   egg
1   teaspoon cold water

Combine flour, salt and sugar. Cut in butter and shortening until crumbly. Add water; form a firm ball. Knead dough briefly to uniformly mix butter. Wrap in plastic wrap and refrigerate at least one hour before rolling. Combine cheese, nuts and egg. Add seasonings to taste. Preheat oven to 350°. Roll out chilled dough to 3/16-inch thickness. Trim to 12-inch square. Transfer to baking sheet. Spread half of dough with cheese nut filling, leaving a 1-inch margin around edge. Moisten edges lightly with cold water. Turn top of dough over filling. Crimp edges to seal. In separate bowl, beat 1 egg with 1 teaspoon cold water and lightly brush turnover with this egg glaze. Cut parallel slashes completely through top layer of dough, ¾ inches apart. Bake for 30 minutes, or until golden brown. Serve warm.

Susan Braziel
Cape Elizabeth, Maine

Cheese Krispies

"My grandmother loved cheese and crunchy things. This was one of her favorite appetizers. When I visited her, I would make up a supply of them so we could have as many as we wanted."

Preparation Time: 1 hour

Baking Time: 15 minutes

5 dozen

1	stick margarine
1	cup grated sharp cheddar cheese
1	cup flour
1	cup Rice Krispies
¼	teaspoon salt
½-1	teaspoon Tabasco sauce

Preheat oven to 350°. Let margarine and cheese come to room temperature. Blend well. Mix with other ingredients. Pinch off marble sized bits. Place on lightly greased baking sheet. Bake for 15 minutes. These freeze well.

Elizabeth Hatcher
Boulder, Colorado

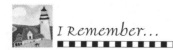

Hot Mushroom Turnovers

Preparation Time: 2 hours

2½ to 3 dozen

1   8-ounce package cream cheese, softened
1½ cups flour
1   stick butter or margarine
8   ounces mushrooms, minced
½   small to medium onion, minced
¼   cup sour cream
½   teaspoon salt
¼   teaspoon dried thyme
2   tablespoons flour
1   egg, beaten

Beat cream cheese, flour and butter together; wrap and refrigerate 1 hour. Preheat oven to 450°. Sauté mushrooms and onions together until tender. Add remaining ingredients, except egg. Roll out cream cheese dough (½ at a time, to save space) ⅛-inch thick. Cut into 2¾-inch rounds. Place 1 teaspoon mushroom filling on each round. Brush edges with egg; fold over and seal. Brush top with egg. Prick tops with fork. Bake on ungreased cookie sheet for 12 to 14 minutes. May be prepared ahead and frozen to bake later.

Hattie Cavanaugh
Bethel, Maine

Tester's Note: This is a winner—the subtle taste of the thyme really adds to the flavor! It is well worth the preparation time for any special occasion.

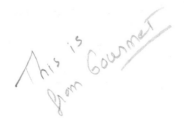

Breads

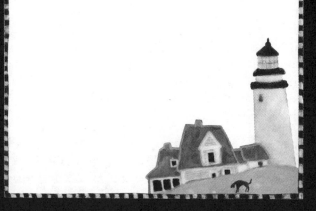

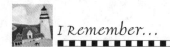

Blueberry Muffins

"Crispy on the outside but soft in the middle."

Preparation Time: 20 minutes

Baking Time: 25 to 30 minutes

1 dozen muffins

1	stick margarine or butter
1¼	cups sugar
2	eggs (or 3 egg whites)
½	cup milk
2	cups flour
2	teaspoons baking powder
½	teaspoon salt
2½	cups blueberries

Preheat oven to 375°. Cream margarine and sugar until fluffy.
Add eggs one at a time. Mix until well blended. Add dry
ingredients, alternating with milk, to the creamed mixture.
Add ½ cup blueberries and stir by hand. Add rest of berries
and fold in. Pile batter high in lined muffin pans. Bake for 25 to
30 minutes. Cool 15 minutes before removing from pan.

Deanne Bailey
Mechanicsville, Virginia

Six Week Bran Muffins

"This recipe comes from a bake sale at Phippsburg 30 to 35 years ago."

Preparation Time: 10 minutes

Baking Time: 15 to 20 minutes

More than 2 dozen muffins

1	15-ounce box raisin bran
5	cups flour
3	cups sugar
5	teaspoons baking soda
1	quart buttermilk
1	cup vegetable oil
4	eggs

Preheat oven to 400°. Mix dry ingredients together in very large bowl. First use spoon to get dry ingredients well blended; then use hands to break up bran flakes a bit. Make well in center and add rest of ingredients and mix until well blended. Spoon into greased or lined muffin pans and bake for 15 to 20 minutes until brown. Remaining batter can be stored in refrigerator in tight container for up to 6 weeks. Bake as needed.

Jean Vetter
Chestertown, New York

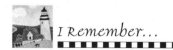

Pumpkin Muffins

"I made these muffins in a restaurant where I used to cook. My mom loved them and I would make them when she and dad would go cruising up the coast. They would be stored in the bow where it would become very warm. In the morning my mom would row to the other boats and serve the muffins. Everyone was surprised, not only at the hot muffins made on the boat, but also because she did not have a reputation as a cook."

Preparation Time: 30 minutes

Baking Time: 25 to 30 minutes

2 dozen muffins

1	stick butter or margarine
1½	cups sugar
2	eggs
1	cup pumpkin purée
1⅔	cups flour
½	teaspoon baking powder
1	teaspoon baking soda
½	teaspoon salt
¼	teaspoon ground cloves
1	teaspoon cinnamon
½	teaspoon nutmeg

Preheat oven to 350°. Cream butter and sugar. Beat in eggs. Beat in pumpkin purée. Mix dry ingredients and add to mixture. Beat well. Fill well-greased muffin tins ¾ full. Bake for 25 to 30 minutes.

Sally Sewall
South Portland, Maine

Apple Raisin Muffins

"This recipe was given to me by a friend. The muffins are delicious and moist and I make them all the time. When I give them away, everyone wants the recipe."

Preparation Time: 20 minutes

20 to 25 minutes

1 dozen

¾	cup vegetable oil
1	cup sugar
2	eggs
1	teaspoon vanilla
2	cups flour
¾	teaspoon soda
¾	teaspoon cinnamon
½	teaspoon salt
1½	cups diced apples
½	cup raisins
½	cup walnuts, chopped

Preheat oven to 400°. Lightly grease muffin tins. Beat oil and sugar 2 minutes. Add eggs and vanilla and beat 1 minute. In another bowl, stir flour, baking soda, cinnamon and salt. Add these dry ingredients to oil mixture, stirring just to combine. Stir in apples, raisins and walnuts. Bake 20 to 25 minutes for regular sized muffins (15 to 16 minutes for mini muffins).

Peggy Thompson
South Portland, Maine

Cranberry Apple Muffins

Preparation Time: 15 minutes

Baking Time: 25 minutes

1 dozen

2 cups flour
2 teaspoons baking powder
¾ cup sugar, divided
½ teaspoon salt
3 tablespoons unsalted butter, melted and cooled
1 egg, beaten
½ cup buttermilk
½ cup apple cider
1 cup chopped cranberries
1 cup chopped apples

Preheat oven to 400°. Grease muffin tins. Sift flour, baking powder, ¼ cup sugar and salt into bowl. Whisk cooled butter together with egg, buttermilk and cider. Add this mixture to dry ingredients, stirring only enough to mix. Batter should be stiff. Fold cranberries and apples into batter and fill muffin cups ⅔ full. Sprinkle an additional teaspoon of sugar over each muffin. Bake 20 to 25 minutes, or until muffins test clean in center. Turn out on rack to cool.

Georgina Burt
Cape Elizabeth, Maine

Tester's Notes: If fresh cranberries are not available, you may use dried. Apple juice may be substituted for cider.

Banana Chocolate Chip Muffins

"These muffins, baked in small tins and frozen, make a nice travel treat for children."

Preparation Time: 25 minutes

Baking Time: 20 to 25 minutes

1 dozen

3½ small ripe bananas, mashed
1   cup sugar
1   cup oil
1   teaspoon vanilla
2   eggs, slightly beaten
½   cup uncooked quick oatmeal
2   cups flour
¾   tablespoon baking powder
⅛   teaspoon salt
1   tablespoon chocolate powdered drink mix (optional)
1   cup chocolate chips

Preheat oven to 350°. Combine sugar, oil and vanilla. Add eggs. Mix oatmeal, flour, baking powder, salt and powdered drink mix in small bowl and add, alternating with mashed bananas. Stir in chips. Pour into slightly greased muffin tins and bake for 20 to 25 minutes. Remove immediately from tins.

Grace Reny
Scarborough, Maine

French Breakfast Muffins

Preparation Time: 30 minutes

Baking Time: 25 minutes

1 to 2 dozen muffins

⅓   cup oil
½   cup sugar
1   egg
1½ cups flour
1½ teaspoons baking powder
½   teaspoon salt
¼   teaspoon nutmeg
½   cup milk

Topping
½   cup sugar
1   teaspoon cinnamon
1   stick melted butter or margarine

Preheat oven to 350°. Grease muffin pans. Mix oil, sugar and egg together. Add remaining ingredients and stir just until moistened. Pour in muffin pan and bake 25 minutes or until golden. While still hot, first roll in melted butter or margarine and then in cinnamon-sugar mixture. Serve warm.

Penny Porter
Glenburn, Maine

Blueberry Scone Cake

"It was a tradition to bring all ingredients below (dry ones premixed) to camp and then put together at the last minute so the cake would be hot for the Brown family gathering. This scone cake, from "Brownie" Schrumpf's cookbook, was published by the "Bangor Daily News." My aunt continued her weekly column of recipes until she was 90 years old."

Preparation Time: 20 minutes

Baking Time: 30 to 35 minutes

9 generous servings

2	cups sifted all-purpose flour
½	cup sugar
2	teaspoons baking powder
½	teaspoon baking soda
½	teaspoon salt
½	cup shortening, margarine or butter
2	eggs, beaten
½	cup sour milk or buttermilk
1½	cups fresh, frozen or canned blueberries

Preheat oven to 375°. Mix and sift the dry ingredients into a bowl; cut in shortening as for biscuits. Mix sour milk or buttermilk and beaten eggs; add to dry ingredients. Mix to form a soft dough. (It may take 2 or 3 more tablespoons of sour milk, according to size of eggs.) Stir in blueberries. If using canned blueberries, drain, rinse and then drain again. Frozen berries do not need to be defrosted. Bake in a greased 9x9-inch pan for 30 to 35 minutes. Serve hot or split and toast, if cold.

Joan Dow Scott for Mildred Brown Schrumpf
Bangor, Maine

Tester's Note: Can pre-mix dry ingredients the night before.

cranberry coffee cake

Preparation Time: 35 minutes

Baking Time: 55 minutes

12 to 16 servings

1   stick margarine or butter
1   cup sugar
2   eggs
2   cups sifted flour
1   teaspoon baking soda
½   teaspoon salt
1   cup sour cream
1   teaspoon almond extract
1   can whole cranberry sauce
½   cup chopped walnuts

Glaze
¾   cup confectioners' sugar
1   tablespoon warm water
⅓   teaspoon almond flavoring

Preheat oven to 350°. Grease and flour angel cake pan. Cream together margarine or butter, sugar and eggs. Add sifted flour, soda and salt, alternating with sour cream and almond extract. Beat batter until smooth and creamy. Pour half batter in pan and top with ½ of the cranberries. Add rest of batter and cover with remaining cranberries. Top off with chopped walnuts. Bake for 55 minutes. Cool 5 to 10 minutes and remove from pan, nut side up, and glaze.

Veronica Sheehan
Saco, Maine

cinnamon swirl coffee cake

"This recipe was given to me 18 years ago by Vera Brown, a neighbor who lived across from Orono Commons. Two years ago she became a resident at Orono Commons. It gave her so much happiness to know how many times I had given the recipe to others and how they loved the coffee cake."

Preparation Time: 20 minutes

Baking Time: 40 minutes

16 servings

1	stick margarine or butter, melted
1	cup sugar
1	teaspoon vanilla
2	eggs
2	cups flour
1	teaspoon baking powder
1	teaspoon baking soda
1	cup sour cream

Cinnamon Mixture

¾	cup sugar
1	teaspoon cinnamon

Preheat oven to 350°. Grease angel or bundt cake pan. In large bowl, cream sugar and margarine or butter. Add vanilla and eggs. Mix well. Combine flour, baking powder and baking soda. Add flour mixture, alternating with sour cream. Spread ½ dough in greased pan. Add layer of cinnamon sugar, then drop remaining dough (by tablespoons) around pan. Do not smooth this layer at all. Add sprinkle of cinnamon and sugar on top. Bake for 40 minutes. Cool for 15 minutes and invert onto large plate and invert again.

Orono Commons-Diane Tinkham
Orono, Maine

All-Bran Brown Bread

"This shiny topped bread is especially good when served with baked beans."

Preparation Time: 15 minutes

Baking Time: 25 minutes

1 8x8-inch pan

1	cup flour, sifted
1	teaspoon baking soda
½	teaspoon salt
2	tablespoons shortening or corn oil
1	cup bran cereal
¾	cup hot water
½	cup molasses
1	egg
½	cup seedless raisins

Preheat oven to 350°. Mix flour with soda and salt in bowl. Set aside. Combine shortening or corn oil and bran cereal in bowl. Add hot water, molasses, and flour mixture, stirring after each addition. Add egg. Stir in raisins. Pour batter into greased 8x8-inch pan and bake for 25 minutes. Cool 10 minutes and remove from pan.

Inez M. Farrell
Brewer, Maine

True Irish Soda Bread

"When my grandmother immigrated to America, she brought this recipe with her. "Gram" always baked this in a large cast iron skillet."

Preparation Time: 30 to 45 minutes

Baking Time: 1 hour 10 minutes

1 large loaf

2   cups raisins
4   cups sifted flour
1   teaspoon baking soda
1   teaspoon baking powder
1   teaspoon salt
½   cup sugar
⅓   cup caraway seeds
⅓   cup shortening
1⅓ cups buttermilk
2   eggs

Topping
¼   cup milk
¼   cup water

Preheat oven to 375°. Put raisins in small pan and add enough water to cover. Heat on very low heat for 30 minutes until plump. Drain well and set aside. Sift dry ingredients into large bowl. Stir in caraway seeds. Cut shortening in with knife until it resembles cornmeal. Combine buttermilk and eggs and stir into flaky mixture. Add raisins and stir. (Dough will be sticky.) Grease 10-inch round low sided pan. (Use square pan if needed.) Knead dough a few times and turn into greased baking dish. Shape bread in round pan so that the center of loaf is slightly higher than sides. Dip a sharp knife in butter or shortening just to coat and cut a cross into dough about ¼ to ½-inch deep. The cross is not just a religious symbol. Its purpose is to prevent loaf from splitting. It is also easier to divide after it is baked. Dilute a small amount of milk with water and brush onto top of loaf. Bake for 1 hour and 10 minutes or until golden brown and firm when tapped.

Dr. Jim Donahue
Cumberland, Maine

Banana Bread

Preparation Time: 20 minutes

Baking Time: 1 hour

2 4½x8½-inch loaves

2   cups flour
¾   teaspoon baking soda
½   teaspoon baking powder
¼   teaspoon salt
¼   teaspoon cinnamon
1   stick butter, softened
1½ cups sugar
2   eggs
2   ripe bananas, mashed
¼   cup milk
1   cup chopped nuts (optional)

Preheat oven to 325°. Stir first 5 ingredients in bowl. In separate bowl, cream butter and sugar. Beat in 2 eggs, one at a time to creamed mixture. Add bananas and milk. Beat. Add dry ingredients and mix well. Stir in nuts. Divide into 2 greased loaf pans. Bake for 1 hour, or until toothpick comes out clean.

Elaine Smith
Cape Elizabeth, Maine

Strawberry Bread

Preparation Time: 20 minutes

Baking Time: 1 hour

2 9x5-inch loaves

2	10-ounce packages whole frozen strawberries (not in syrup)
4	eggs
1½	cups oil
3	cups flour
2	cups sugar
3	teaspoons cinnamon
1	teaspoon baking soda
1	teaspoon salt
1	cup chopped nuts

Preheat oven to 350°. Thaw strawberries. Grease and flour 2 9x5-inch loaf pans. Mix strawberries, eggs and oil. Combine flour, sugar, cinnamon, baking soda, salt and nuts. Add the berry mixture to the dry ingredients. Stir until blended. Pour into loaf pans. Bake for at least 1 hour, or until toothpick tests clean in middle of loaf. Cool in pans for 10 minutes. Remove and cool on rack. These loaves can be frozen.

Kathy Crispin
Scarborough, Maine

Tester's Note: This bread is good for dessert served with fruit.

Lemon Zucchini Tea Bread

"This was a favorite of my mother and father. When my mother could no longer cook, my father took over. Though cooking was not a familiar task, my father mastered several recipes, this one, especially. Perhaps it was because he would never throw anything away, including the "ball-bat" zucchinis he grew in his garden, which no one would eat. So he made loaves upon loaves of bread for us and the neighbors."

Preparation Time: 45 to 60 minutes

Baking time: 35 minutes

2 4x8-inch loaves

3½ cups flour, sifted
¾ teaspoon baking powder
1½ teaspoons baking soda
1½ teaspoons salt
2 teaspoons lemon peel
2 cups sugar
1 cup oil
1 teaspoon vanilla
4 eggs
2 cups zucchini, grated medium to fine
1 cup chopped walnuts
1 cup raisins

Preheat oven to 350°. Mix first 5 ingredients together. In large bowl, beat sugar, oil and vanilla. Beat in eggs, one at a time. Add dry ingredients, alternating with zucchini. Stir in nuts and raisins. Pour into two slightly oiled 4x8-inch pans. Bake for 35 minutes or until toothpick comes out clean. Loosen sides; remove and cool on racks.

Susan Grondin
Raymond, Maine

Lemon Bread

"Traditionally, my Delaware cousins and I have exchanged recipes and food by mail, especially during the holidays. This is a favorite that can be made ahead, stays moist, freezes well and can go through the mail."

Preparation Time: 30 minutes

Baking Time: 1 hour

1 9½x5½-inch loaf or 3 small loaves

⅓ cup melted butter
1 cup sugar
2 eggs
1½ cups flour, sifted
1 teaspoon baking powder
1 teaspoon salt
½ cup milk
Grated rind of 1 lemon
½ cup chopped nuts (almonds preferred)
¼ teaspoon almond extract

Concentrate
Juice of ½ lemon
¼ cup sugar

Preheat oven to 325°. Grease and flour loaf pan. Combine butter and sugar. Beat in eggs. Sift dry ingredients together and add to above, alternating with milk. Fold in lemon rind, chopped nuts and almond extract. Pour into loaf pan and bake for about an hour or until toothpick comes out clean. Remove immediately from pan. While still hot, drip lemon/sugar concentrate over top. Do not eat for 24 hours to allow concentrate to be absorbed into bread.

Connie Korda
Falmouth, Maine

Pumpkin Mincemeat Bread

Preparation Time: 30 minutes

Baking Time: 60 to 70 minutes

2 9x5-inch loaves or 4 small loaves

3½ cups flour
1½ cups white sugar
2   teaspoons pumpkin pie spice
2   teaspoons baking soda
1½ teaspoons salt
1½ cups brown sugar
4   eggs, slightly beaten
1   cup salad oil
2   cups mashed cooked pumpkin
1   cup mincemeat
1   cup chopped nuts

Preheat oven to 350°. In large bowl, sift flour, white sugar, pumpkin pie spice, baking soda and salt. Mix in brown sugar. Make a well in center and add eggs, oil and pumpkin. Beat at low speed until blended; then beat at medium speed, about 3 minutes. Stir in mincemeat and nuts. Pour into 2 9x5-inch loaf pans or 4 small ones. Bake for 60 to 70 minutes, or until toothpick comes out clean. Cool on rack.

Market Square Health Care Center
South Paris, Maine

Easy Cinnamon Rolls

"Be sure to have copies of this recipe to give to your friends after they have sampled these rolls. They always ask!"

Preparation Time: 10 minutes

Baking Time: 20 minutes

16 rolls

½   cup brown sugar
½   stick plus 2 tablespoons butter or margarine, melted, divided
1   tablespoon water
1   cup chopped walnuts, divided
1   teaspoon cinnamon
½   cup white sugar
2   cans refrigerated biscuits (8 biscuits in each can)

Preheat oven to 400°. Sprinkle brown sugar in bundt pan. Add 2 tablespoons melted margarine or butter and add water. Sprinkle in ½ cup walnuts. Mix cinnamon and white sugar together in small bowl. Separate biscuits; then dip each one in the remaining melted butter or margarine, then in sugar and cinnamon mixture. Stand side by side in Bundt pan. Sprinkle remaining walnuts between each biscuit. Bake for 20 minutes.

Kay H. Marstaller
Camden, Maine

Nanny Neil's Oatmeal Bread

"This recipe came from my husband's Nova Scotian great grandmother. She was a great cook and I was not. So I made this bread often with hopes of gaining her approval. Consequently, all our children, sister, nieces and even grandchildren make this bread. The smell, itself, stirs memories for all of us."

Preparation Time: 30 minutes

Baking Time: 30 minutes

4 loaves

2	cups regular oatmeal
1	tablespoon salt
2	tablespoons butter
1	cup molasses
4	cups boiling water
1	yeast cake or 1 package dry yeast
8-10	cups flour (unbleached is best)
	Salad oil
	Butter, melted

Pour boiling water over oatmeal, salt, butter, and molasses in a very large mixing bowl. Allow to cool to lukewarm. Add yeast and mix. Add 2 cups flour at a time, until consistency is thick enough to turn out on floured board without sticking. Knead, adding more flour, if necessary, until smooth and elastic. Form into a ball and place in a greased bowl. Oil top of dough with salad oil, cover with towel and put in warm place to rise. When doubled, punch down and divide dough into 4 equal parts. Let rest for 10 minutes. Form into 4 loaves and place in greased bread pans. Allow to rise, about 2 hours. Preheat oven to 375°. Bake for 10 minutes then reduce to 350° for 20 minutes. Remove from oven and brush tops with butter. Remove from pans.

Jean Baxter
Portland, Maine

My Easiest Bread Recipe

Preparation Time: 30 minutes

Baking Time: 30 minutes

2 9x5-inch loaves

2½ cups warm water	5 cups flour
1 package rapid-rise yeast	1 teaspoon salt
2 tablespoons oil	Butter or margarine
2 tablespoons sugar	

Combine warm water and yeast. Add oil and sugar and mix together. Add salt and 4 cups flour to form ball. Turn onto floured surface. Knead in 1 cup of flour until smooth. Add more flour if necessary. Put dough in greased bowl. Cover and let rise until double. Cut dough in half and roll each half on floured surface. Roll up like jelly rolls and put in greased loaf pans. Cover and let rise. Preheat oven to 350°. Bake for 30 minutes; never longer. Remove from pans immediately. Brush hot bread with butter or margarine.

Annette Austin
Rumford, Maine

Theresa's Bread

Preparation Time: 15 minutes to mix; 2 hours to rise

Baking Time: 40 to 45 minutes

2 long French loaves or 4 short loaves

1½ tablespoons yeast	1 cup milk
½ cup water	2 teaspoons salt
Pinch of sugar	3 heaping teaspoons solid
4 plus cups flour	shortening

Mix yeast, ¼ cup water, sugar and a pinch of flour and let yeast "proof". In large bowl, mix well 4 cups flour, milk, ¼ cup water, salt and shortening, adding more flour when necessary. Turn dough onto floured surface and knead until dough feels elastic – about 3 to 4 minutes. Place in greased bowl and let rise until double in bulk. Punch dough down, turn onto floured surface and divide into 2 or 4 equal portions. Roll dough with palms, sliding hands gradually towards the ends to lengthen into French-style loaves. Place in French loaf pans. Slash top of each loaf 2 or 3 times with sharp knife or razor blade. Let rise again to double in bulk. Preheat oven to 400°. Bake for 20 minutes. Reduce heat to 350° and bake for 20 to 25 minutes longer.

Sybil Riemensnider
South Portland, Maine

Refrigerator Rolls

"I come from a large family. All of our gatherings are organized so that each family takes responsibility for bringing different parts of the meal. My mother's permanent assignment is to bring yeast rolls. My mother and her companion, Ervin, prepare a triple batch (6 dozen) and bring them covered with dish towels, ready to pop in the oven. The tradition is to bake 3 dozen immediately and eat them as hors d'oeuvres while everything else is being prepared."

Preparation Time: 30 minutes

Baking Time: 12 minutes

24 rolls

1½ cups very warm water
2   packages dry yeast
½   cup sugar
2   teaspoons salt
2   eggs
1   stick butter, softened
½   cup warm mashed potatoes
6½ cups flour

Pour water into large bowl. Sprinkle yeast over water. Add sugar and salt. Stir until dissolved and let stand 3 to 4 minutes. Add eggs, butter, mashed potatoes and 3 cups flour. Beat with mixer. Add 2 cups flour and beat with spoon. Add remaining 1½ cups flour and knead with hands until dough is smooth and stiff. Brush top with melted butter; cover with wax paper and dish towel. Let rise in refrigerator 2 hours or until double in size. Punch down dough. Cover; refrigerate. Dough can be refrigerated from 1 to 3 days; however, dough must be punched down once a day. About 2 hours before serving, remove dough from refrigerator. Lightly grease muffin tins. To shape rolls: turn dough onto floured board. Cut into 3 equal pieces, cutting these pieces in half. Continue to halve the resulting pieces of dough until you have 96 small pieces. Place 3 pieces in each muffin cup to form a clover shaped roll. Let rise. Preheat oven to 400°. Brush with butter or margarine before baking. Bake for 12 minutes.

Liz Weaver
Cape Elizabeth, Maine

Gougère

Preparation Time: 20 to 30 minutes

Baking Time: 35 to 45 minutes

8 to 10 servings

1	cup flour
⅔	cup Swiss or Gruyère cheese, shredded, divided
½	teaspoon dry mustard
	Vinegar
½	stick butter
⅔	cup water
½	teaspoon salt
5	eggs

Measure flour into cup and set near stove. Measure out ¼ cup cheese
and reserve for topping. Moisten mustard with splash of vinegar and
set aside. Cut butter into 4 pieces and put in saucepan with water and
salt. Bring to boil, stirring occasionally. Butter should melt before boil
is reached. As soon as boil is reached, lower heat to simmer and add
flour all at once. Stir vigorously with wooden spoon until all flour is
absorbed and thick dough results. Use spoon to mash dough against
bottom and sides of pan for 1 to 2 minutes. Remove pan from heat
and let stand for 3 minutes. Place dough in processor bowl with steel
blade and blend for 10 to 15 seconds. With motor running, add 4
eggs, one at a time, through tube. Add remaining cheese and
mustard/vinegar mixture; process until dough is smooth and shiny
(about 25 to 30 seconds). Mixture will be very thick. (Dough can be
used immediately, or refrigerated, covered, for 1 to 2 days.) When
ready to bake, preheat oven to 375°. Drop dough from tablespoon on
greased baking sheet to form a circle of adjacent mounds. Lightly
beat remaining egg and brush on dough. Sprinkle with reserved
cheese and bake until puffed, browned and dry, 35 to 45 minutes.
Best served warm from the oven.

Kathleen Leslie
Cape Elizabeth, Maine

**Note: Gougère is similar in texture to a popover or a savory cream
puff. It's so easy to make the dough ahead and bake at the last
minute. We love it served with soups or as an addition to meals of
all kinds. The dough may also be dropped as smaller individual
puffs to serve as hors d'oeuvres, with or without a filling.**

Sticky Buns

Preparation Time: 30 minutes

Baking Time: 20 minutes

20 buns

1	package dry yeast
½	cup warm water
1	egg white, slightly beaten
2	cups flour
1	tablespoon sugar
¼	cup softened butter
1	teaspoon cinnamon

Filling

½	cup sugar
1	teaspoon cinnamon

Sticky Bun Topping

⅔	cup brown sugar
¼	cup butter
2	tablespoons light corn syrup
1	cup chopped pecans

Add yeast dissolved in warm water to slightly beaten egg white. Let sit. Blend flour, sugar, butter and cinnamon together. Mix together flour mixture and yeast mixture. Turn out on floured surface and knead until smooth. More water or flour may be needed. Cover and put in warm place for 20 to 30 minutes. Turn dough out on floured board and roll into rectangle. Sprinkle with cinnamon and sugar mixture. Roll up like a jelly roll and cut into 1-inch slices. While dough is rising, put brown sugar, butter and corn syrup in small sauce pan and cook until sugar is dissolved. Add pecans. Distribute evenly in muffin tins. Add cut dough to muffin tin and put in a cold oven to rise for 20 minutes. Remove. Turn on oven to 325°. When ready bake for about 20 minutes. Remove muffin tins from oven and turn upside down. Serve warm.

Tonia Nadzo Medd
Peaks Island, Maine

Dansk Jule Kage
(Danish Christmas Bread)

"Christmas gift exchange in Denmark always happens on Christmas Eve. In keeping with American tradition, however, we exchange on Christmas morning before breakfast. Serving the Jule Kage while opening gifts has been a special tradition in my family."

Preparation Time: 45 minutes plus rising time

Baking Time: 30 to 35 minutes

2 round loaves

1	stick butter
½	cup milk
1	package dry yeast
½	cup warm water
¼	cup sugar
1	teaspoon salt
1	cup raisins
¾	cup chopped candied fruit, divided
½	teaspoon cardamom
½	cup almonds
1	slightly beaten egg (reserve 1 tablespoon)
3½-4	cups flour

Frosting

1	cup sifted powdered sugar
2	drops almond extract
1-2	tablespoons light cream to make spreading consistency

Heat butter and milk until butter melts. Cool to lukewarm. Soften yeast in warm water in mixing bowl. Stir in sugar, salt, raisins, candied fruit (reserve a little for topping), cardamom, almonds, egg and milk mixture. Gradually add flour to form stiff dough. Let rise in warm place 1½ to 2 hours. Turn out onto floured board. Toss lightly until coated with flour and not sticky. Cut dough in half, shape into 2 round loaves and place on greased baking sheet or in 2 8-inch round pans. Let rise 1 hour. Preheat oven to 350°. Bake in oven for 30 to 35 minutes. Brush loaves with reserved egg. Cool. At this point, loaves can be wrapped and frozen. Frost and decorate with reserved candied fruit.

Sarah Pedersen deDoes
Portland, Maine

Easter Bread

"This recipe was prepared by my grandmother, Maria Teresa Salatino, of Rumford, Maine, every year at Easter time. I remember my grandmother, who is under 5 feet tall, kerchief in her hair, wearing a long apron and standing over a very large metal pan filled with risen dough. Entering her kitchen, smelling the wonderful aroma of freshly baked Easter bread, dripping with frosting and sprinkles, was heaven. She would make one for each of her 11 children and numerous grandchildren. You couldn't wait to taste it."

Preparation Time: 1 hour

Baking Time: 30 minutes to 1 hour

5 loaves

2	cups warm water
1	yeast cake
1½	cups butter or margarine, melted and cooled
1½	cups sugar
1	dozen eggs
1	1-ounce bottle lemon extract
8	cups flour

Glaze

1	cup powdered sugar
6-8	teaspoons milk
	Candy sprinkles

In large bowl, dissolve yeast in water. Blend in butter or margarine, sugar and eggs. Using mixer, add lemon extract and 1 cup flour until moistened. Stir in rest of flour by hand making a soft, sticky batter. It may be necessary to add more flour depending on size of eggs. Turn out onto floured surface and knead until smooth. Put in large bowl and let rise until double. Punch down. Divide dough in 15 equal pieces and roll each piece out like a rope. Take 3 ropes and braid together, shaping into a round cake pan. Pinch ends together. Let rise again to top of pan. Preheat oven to 300°. Bake until done between 30 minutes to 1 hour. Bread should be light, not heavy, and golden brown in color. If bread cooks too fast, it will not be cooked on inside. When cool, bread may be frosted and decorated with tiny candy sprinkles. To make glaze: combine powdered sugar and milk until smooth. This bread is best served toasted under the broiler with butter.

Debra Soubble
Scarborough, Maine

Tester's Note: May add raisins to batter. Stir raisins in with flour.

Steve's Old Fashioned Donuts

"Steve makes these donuts better than anyone I know. He searched for the perfect donut and seems to have found it. He is always happy to make the donuts for fund raisers and I am usually on the clean up detail. Steve is a great cook, but a messy one."

Preparation Time: 1 hour 30 minutes

15 to 20 donuts

3½-4	cups flour
3	teaspoons baking powder
1	teaspoon salt
½	teaspoon cinnamon
¼	teaspoon nutmeg
⅛	teaspoon ground cloves
2	large eggs
⅔	cup sugar
1	cup milk
5	tablespoons melted margarine or butter
1	teaspoon vanilla
	Oil, enough for deep frying

Combine flour, baking powder, salt and spices in large mixing bowl. In separate bowl, beat eggs and sugar with electric beater. Beat on high until thick and pale yellow. Add milk, butter or margarine and vanilla. On low speed, add dry ingredients. Turn out onto floured surface and knead, adding more flour as needed to form a soft dough. Let rest for 30 minutes. Heat oil to 370°. Roll out, cut and fry, turning with tongs when side is browned. Continue until both sides are browned. Drain on paper bag and sprinkle with sugar, cinnamon/sugar or enjoy plain.

Cheri Alexander
Boothbay, Maine

chocolate Sugared Donuts

"This is my mother and father's famous chocolate sugared donuts recipe. They were owners of the Chisholm Pastry Shop in Chisholm where they served the mill workers, as well as the public of 2 towns, for 32 years. They also catered weddings, funerals and town events. It was a family business with 6 children and grandchildren all working to make it such a success. Our mother, Dorothy Therrien, diagnosed with Alzheimer's at age 60, was the most wonderful cook."

Preparation Time: 45 minutes

3 dozen

5	eggs
1	pound plus 4 ounces sugar
1	quart milk
2	ounces melted shortening
3	pounds plus 4 ounces flour
2½	ounces baking powder
3	ounces cocoa
1	ounce salt
	Oil, enough for deep frying
	Sugar, for coating donuts

Heat oil to 375°. Beat eggs and sugar until light; add milk and cooled shortening. Sift flour, baking powder, cocoa and salt and add, mixing until smooth. Roll ⅜-inch thick on lightly floured surface. Cut out donuts, using floured cutter. Fry, turning when side is done. Drain on paper towel. Cool and roll in sugar.

The Therrien Children
Jay, Maine

Potato Donuts

"Although these donuts are not on the health food list, they are tasty and moist. They also keep longer than other donuts and they freeze well. I have tried several shortenings for frying but prefer using lard. Instant potato flakes work well to make the mashed potatoes. This recipe is my mother's old standby."

Preparation Time: 45 minutes

Frying Time: 3 minutes

2 dozen

2   eggs
2   tablespoons melted shortening
1¼   cups sugar
1   cup buttermilk
2   teaspoons baking soda, divided
1   cup mashed potatoes
1   tablespoon vanilla
2   teaspoons cream of tartar
1   teaspoon salt
1   teaspoon nutmeg, rounded
    Pinch of ginger
4   cups flour
4   pounds lard (or other shortening), for frying

Mix eggs, melted shortening, sugar and buttermilk to which 1 teaspoon of baking soda has been added. Add mashed potatoes and vanilla. Sift remaining dry ingredients together and stir into mixture 1 cup at a time. Refrigerate overnight or longer before frying or dough will be too soft to handle. Roll lightly to about ¼-inch thick. Cut, using floured cutter, and fry in 340° to 350° shortening, about 1½ minutes per side. Donuts should rise immediately. Prick each donut lightly several times.

Christine Wright
East Vassalboro, Maine

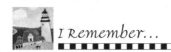

Dog Bones

"We have made a special activity for our residents with this recipe. We make and donate the dog bones to a local animal shelter; or we bake them a day or two before the pet therapy dogs come in so that the residents can give each dog a treat."

Preparation Time: 20 minutes

Baking Time: 40 minutes

36 3-inch bones

2	cups whole wheat flour
2	cups white flour
2	eggs
1	cup dry milk
1	cup wheat germ
3	tablespoons molasses
1	tablespoon minced garlic
1	cup shortening
	Water

Preheat oven to 300°. Mix all ingredients together, adding water, as necessary, until the consistency of bread dough. Knead 2 to 3 minutes. Roll out onto a floured surface ½-inch thick. Use cookie cutters (dog bone shape or any shape desired) and cut out dough. Place on nonstick or greased cookie sheet. Bake for about 40 minutes. Let cool until hard.

Lynne Whitney, Norway Rehabilitation and Living Center Norway, Maine

Breakfast & Brunch

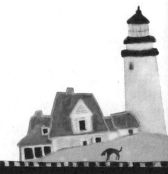

Madelyn's Salmon Quiche

"This recipe was written by hand on a note pad, dated 1983, by a friend who was a wonderful cook and fellow speech therapist. She's no longer with us, having lost her battle with a brain tumor when she was much too young. Preparing this easy and wonderful quiche always brings me back... and I remember Madelyn."

Preparation Time: 10 minutes

Baking Time: 40 minutes

6 servings

1	9-inch frozen pie shell
½	cup mayonnaise
½	cup milk
2	eggs, beaten
2	tablespoons flour
1	pound can salmon, drained and boned
⅓	cup chopped scallions
1	8-ounce package Jarlsberg (or Swiss) cheese, shredded

Preheat oven to 350°. Blend mayonnaise, milk, eggs and flour. Stir in salmon, cheese and scallions. Pour into pie shell. Bake for 40 minutes until brown and the center is solid. To freeze: Bake 20 minutes. Freeze; finish baking after defrosting.

Vera Berv
Scarborough, Maine

crabmeat Quiche

"A brunch favorite. One daughter likes it cold!"

Preparation Time: 20 to 30 minutes

Baking Time: 55 to 60 minutes

8 servings

3   eggs
1   cup sour cream
½   teaspoon Worcestershire sauce
1   cup shredded Swiss cheese
1   7½-ounce package crabmeat, drained
1   9-inch baked pie shell

Preheat oven to 300°. Combine eggs, sour cream and Worcestershire sauce. Stir in cheese and crabmeat. Pour into pie shell. Bake 55 to 60 minutes. Serve hot.

Elaine Fantle Shimberg
Scarborough, Maine

spinach and cheese Quiche

Preparation Time: 10 minutes

Baking Time: 25 minutes

2 to 3 servings

2   eggs, slightly beaten
1¼ cup cottage cheese
1   10-ounce package frozen spinach, cooked and drained
½   teaspoon salt
¼   teaspoon pepper
4   tablespoons grated cheese

Preheat oven to 350°. Mix together eggs, cottage cheese, salt, pepper and 2 tablespoons cheese. Blend in spinach. Put mixture in greased 9-inch pie plate. Sprinkle with rest of cheese. Bake for 25 minutes.

Charlene Ferguson
Yarmouth, Maine

Quiche

"This recipe was given to me many moons ago by one of my housemates on Fire Island, New York. It brings back memories of lots of fun, sun and great summers. It's great as an hors d'oeuvre or as an entrée with a salad. It was a big hit in our restaurant."

Preparation Time: 10 minutes

Baking Time: 65 minutes

4 servings

1	prepared pie shell
3	eggs, beaten
1	cup cream
1	cup grated Swiss cheese
	Salt and pepper to taste
	Dash nutmeg
	Dash cayenne pepper
½	cup additions: spinach, crumbled bacon, shrimp or whatever you want

Preheat oven to 425°. Put eggs in measuring cup and add cream to make 1½ cups. Put egg mixture in bowl and stir in cheese, seasonings and any additions. Pour into pie shell and bake for 15 minutes; reduce heat to 300° and bake for 40 minutes.

Dorothy Almog
Santa Monica, California

For some reason not as good as Julia Child's — almost $too?, maybe

Temp. Time !!!

Tomato Tart

Preparation Time: 30 minutes

Baking Time: 40 minutes

6 servings

1   stick plus 5 tablespoons butter
1¾ cups flour
     Pinch salt
1   egg
2-3 tablespoons mustard
½   pound Gruyère cheese, grated
4-6 medium tomatoes, sliced

Topping
1   clove garlic, minced
1   teaspoon fresh, minced parsley
1   teaspoon fresh minced oregano
1   teaspoon fresh minced basil
¼   cup olive oil

Preheat oven to 400°. In food processor pulse butter and flour
until grainy. Add egg and process until it forms a ball. Press into
bottom and sides of quiche pan. Refrigerate for 1 hour. Rub
mustard on bottom and sides of crust. Sprinkle cheese evenly over
mustard-coated crust. Place tomatoes over cheese, overlapping
slightly. Bake for 40 minutes. For topping, stir together all
ingredients. Dribble topping over tart when done cooking.

Eleanor Goldberg
Portland, Maine

Easy Garden Vegetable Pie

Preparation Time: 20 minutes

Baking Time: 35 to 40 minutes

6 servings

½   cup chopped onion
½   cup chopped green pepper
1   tablespoon butter or oil
2   cups cooked chopped fresh broccoli or fresh cauliflower
1   cup shredded cheddar cheese (about 4 ounces)
3   eggs
1½ cups milk
¾   cup baking mix
1   teaspoon salt (optional)
¼   teaspoon pepper

Preheat oven to 400°. Slightly grease 9-inch pie plate. Sauté onion and green pepper in butter or oil. Mix broccoli, cheese, onion and green pepper in pie plate. Beat together eggs, milk, baking mix, salt and pepper until smooth. Pour over vegetables. Bake for 35 to 40 minutes until golden brown. Let stand 5 minutes before serving.

Marjorie Jamback
Biddeford, Maine

cheddar-spinach pie

"This is a real family favorite and so easy to prepare. It's like a spinach quiche. Wonderful with fish."

Preparation Time: 20 minutes

Baking Time: 40 minutes

8 servings

2	cups shredded, sharp, natural cheddar cheese
2	tablespoons flour
4	eggs, beaten
1	cup milk
¼	teaspoon salt
	Dash pepper
1	10-ounce package frozen chopped spinach, cooked and well drained

Preheat oven to 350°. Toss cheese with flour. Combine eggs, milk and seasonings. Add cheese mixture and spinach to eggs. Mix well. Pour into greased 9-inch pie plate. Bake for 40 minutes.

Sandy Enck
Scarborough, Maine

Sunny Vegetable Strata

"Here's something special for brunch that is delicious, on the light side, and which the vegetarians in the family can enjoy. It must be made the day before, so just pop it in the oven in the morning."

Preparation Time: 1 hour

Baking Time: 50 to 60 minutes

10 to 12 servings

½   pound mushrooms, thinly sliced
3   tablespoons olive oil
2   cups chopped onion
½   cup chopped scallions
2   red peppers, thinly sliced
2   green peppers thinly sliced
9   cups diced Italian bread (1-inch cubes)
2½ cups shredded cheddar cheese
1   cup freshly grated Parmesan cheese
12 eggs
3½ cups milk
3   tablespoons Dijon mustard
    Dash hot pepper sauce
    Salt and pepper to taste

Sauté mushrooms in olive oil until soft. Add onions, scallions and peppers and cook until moisture has evaporated, 10 to 15 minutes. Divide half the bread cubes between 2 buttered 13x9-inch baking dishes. Arrange half the vegetables over the bread cubes. Mix the cheddar and Parmesan cheese together. Sprinkle vegetables with half the cheese mixture. Divide rest of the bread cubes between the baking dishes. Top with remaining vegetables and then cheeses. Whisk together eggs, milk, mustard, hot pepper sauce, salt and pepper. Pour evenly over top of both dishes. Cover and refrigerate overnight. Preheat oven to 350°. Bake for 50 to 60 minutes.

Patricia Noonan
Purchase, New York

Do-Ahead Breakfast Casserole

"I got this recipe from a good friend and I've used it every Christmas morning for the past 4 or 5 years. It's perfect for a hungry family after opening Christmas gifts and it can be cooking while everyone (even the cook) is enjoying the unwrapping. It is delicious with plenty of orange juice (or mimosas) and English muffins."

Preparation Time: 20 minutes

Baking Time: 1 hour

8 to 10 servings

4	slices any kind of bread, cubed
2	cups shredded cheddar cheese
10	eggs, lightly beaten
1	quart milk
1	teaspoon dry mustard
1	teaspoon salt
¼	teaspoon onion powder
	Dash pepper
½	cup sliced mushrooms
1½	pounds ground sausage, cooked and cooled
½	cup chopped tomatoes

Place bread cubes in 9x13-inch baking pan. Mix all other ingredients together and pour over bread. Refrigerate overnight. Preheat oven to 325°. Bake, uncovered, for 1 hour. (Can also be cooked right after assembling.)

Evelyn Bodemer
Andover, Maine

Breakfast Casserole

"I have used this in quantity for a church breakfast with good success. It was nice to prepare it the night before and bake it in the morning. The honey adds a touch of sweetness."

Preparation Time: 20 minutes

Baking Time: 40 to 50 minutes

8 servings

¼	cup margarine
½	pound asparagus, cut into 1-inch pieces
1	medium onion, diced
1	loaf French bread, cubed (about 8 cups)
2	cups shredded cheddar cheese
1	cup cubed ham
1	tablespoon honey
8	large eggs
2½	cups milk
½	teaspoon salt
½	teaspoon pepper

Sauté asparagus and onion in margarine for 3 to 5 minutes. In 9x13x2-inch baking pan layer bread, then ham, 1 cup of cheese and sautéed vegetables. Beat eggs, milk, honey and seasonings together. Pour over layers and top with remaining cup of cheese. Refrigerate overnight. Preheat oven to 350°. Bake for 45 to 50 minutes.

Jane Hards
Camden, Maine

Corn Fritters

"I make these every Easter for brunch."

Preparation Time: 30 minutes

6 large fritters

1   cup flour
1   teaspoon baking powder
1   teaspoon salt
2   eggs
½   cup milk
1   teaspoon vegetable oil
1   cup well drained corn
     Vegetable oil for frying
     Pure maple syrup

Blend dry ingredients together in bowl. Mix eggs, milk and 1 teaspoon oil. Add to dry ingredients and beat until smooth. Stir in corn. Heat oil to 375° in fryer or skillet. Drop by tablespoons into hot fat. Brown on both sides. Drain on paper towel. Serve with maple syrup.

Roberta Conerrette
St. Agatha, Maine

Buttermilk Waffles

"This waffle recipe is from the Charleston, S.C. Junior League 1950 cookbook, and was offered by Miss L.A. Passailaique, who called it 'Miss Adkins' Crisp Buttermilk Waffles'. I don't know either of these ladies; I just know they're the best waffles you will ever taste. I once traded the recipe with our chimney sweep, who cooks his waffles on a wood cookstove in Hancock County, Maine."

Preparation Time: 20 minutes

3 double waffles

¾   cup flour
¼   teaspoon baking soda
¼   teaspoon salt
2   teaspoons baking powder
2   eggs, well beaten
¾   cup (approximately) buttermilk
5   tablespoons cooking oil

Sift together flour, baking soda, salt and baking powder. In a bowl, beat the eggs. Add a portion of the dry mixture to the eggs and then a small amount of buttermilk, mixing well. Alternate adding flour and buttermilk three times until all the flour mixture has been used and the batter is thin. Add cooking oil and stir to blend well. Cook immediately in standard waffle iron.

Harriet H. Price
Portland, Maine

Crêpes

"The family keeps blocks of maple sugar in the freezer so they can enjoy these crêpes year round. It is especially a meal to delight in the spring. My husband, Reno is the best pancake maker of all."

Preparation Time: 15 minutes

2 dozen

1⅔ cups flour
3 teaspoons baking powder
½ teaspoon salt
2 tablespoons sugar
1 egg
1½ cups milk
3 tablespoons shortening, melted
Grated maple sugar block
Butter

Preheat griddle. Sift flour, baking powder and salt together. Beat egg with sugar. Mix milk and shortening with dry ingredients. Add egg mixture and mix well. On griddle, cook on both sides. Serve with maple sugar and butter.

Mrs. Reno Byram
Caribou, Maine

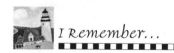

Ployes
(Buckwheat Pancakes)

"This is an Acadian recipe that's been around longer than I have. In the old days it was a daily staple. Today, it's a delicacy. It is delicious with plain butter, syrup, cretons or peanut butter. Some even enjoy them with a hot dog or with ice cream. Remember to roll it after the topping is on it. Serve hot. Leftovers can be warmed up in the microwave on a paper towel."

Preparation Time: 20 to 30 minutes

6 6-inch pancakes

1   cup white flour
1   cup buckwheat flour
2   teaspoons baking powder
    Pinch salt
    Cold water
    Boiling water

Mix dry ingredients together. Add cold water to make a thick heavy paste. Mix very well. Add boiling water to paste gradually, to thin the batter (batter should be quite thin). Spread batter by large spoonfuls (or more for larger pancakes) on to lightly greased griddle and cook on both sides. Top with your favorite topping and roll it to serve.

Diane Voisine
Fort Kent, Maine

Oven French Toast

"Served in a B&B in Indiana. They offer it with maple syrup, but I don't think it needs it."

Preparation Time: 15 minutes

Baking Time: 50 minutes

8 servings

1	loaf (or 12 ounces) of French bread, cut into 1-inch slices
8	large eggs
2	cups milk
2	teaspoons vanilla
½	teaspoon cinnamon
½	teaspoon mace
2	cups half-and-half
½	teaspoon nutmeg

Topping
¾ cup butter, softened
1⅓ cups brown sugar
3 tablespoons dark corn syrup
1⅓ cups coarsely chopped nuts (pecans, hickory or walnuts)

Heavily butter a 13x9x2-inch baking pan. Fill pan with bread to ½ inch of top and set aside. In a blender mix rest of ingredients and pour over bread. Cover and refrigerate overnight. Next morning, preheat oven to 350°. Prepare topping. Mix topping ingredients with fingers until crumbly. Spread topping over bread mixture. Bake approximately 50 minutes until puffed and golden brown. Shield top with foil if browns too quickly.

Helen Riddle
Topsham, Maine

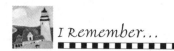
Apricot Strudel

"A trademark recipe that I have made for over 30 years. Wonderful at holidays and parties, or with a cup of coffee and a good book."

Preparation Time: 1 hour

Baking Time: 30 to 35 minutes

4 strudels, each serving 6

2	sticks butter
1	cup sour cream
2	cups sifted flour
1	12-ounce jar apricot preserves
1	8-ounce package coconut
	Powdered sugar

Combine softened butter, sour cream and flour. Divide into 4 parts. Refrigerate overnight. Preheat oven to 350°. Flour each piece; flour pastry cloth and rolling pin cover. Roll one part at a time. Roll very thin. (Dough is rich; use flour to handle.) Gently spread apricot preserves on dough. Sprinkle coconut on preserves. With pastry cloth, flip dough and roll like jelly roll. Place on greased cookie sheet. Bake for 30 to 35 minutes. Dust with powdered sugar.

Fran Lewandowski
South Holland, Illinois

Granola

"Given to me by a friend years ago. It's delicious."

Preparation Time: 15 minutes

Baking Time: 1 hour

8 to 9 cups

Used much less brown sugar. Better than bulk Granola. 1/25/12 Really like This

4	cups rolled oats
2	cups wheat germ
1	cup coarsely chopped nuts (pecans or walnuts)
¾	cup brown sugar
¾	cup cooking oil
2	tablespoons vanilla
⅓	cup water

Preheat oven to 250°. Mix all ingredients together. Spread on lightly greased cookie sheet(s). Cook 1 hour, stirring frequently.

Virginia G. Harvey
Winslow, Maine

Hawaiian Fruit Dip

Preparation Time: 10 minutes

Approximately 3 cups

½	cup sour cream
1	cup milk
1	3½-ounce package instant vanilla pudding
1	8-ounce can crushed pineapple
⅓	cup shredded coconut
	Cantaloupe and other fruits

Mix sour cream, milk and pudding in bowl until smooth.
Add pineapple and coconut and mix to combine. Refrigerate
30 minutes before serving. To serve fill a cantaloupe half with dip
and surround with watermelon, bananas, grapes, strawberries, etc.

Joni Hanson
Westbrook, Maine

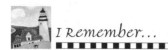

Brown Sugar Syrup for Pancakes and Waffles

Preparation Time: 15 minutes

2 quarts

2   pounds brown sugar
2   pounds granulated sugar
⅓   cup corn syrup
1   quart water
1½ ounces butter or margarine
½   teaspoon maple flavoring (optional)

Combine all ingredients except maple flavoring. Stir and heat until sugar is dissolved. Add maple flavoring, if desired.

Gloria Gove
Norway, Maine

Apricot-Cranberry Conserve

"I usually serve this at Easter with baked ham - delicious!"

Preparation Time: 15 minutes

2½ to 3 cups

1	cup water
¾	cup sugar
2	cups fresh cranberries
½	cup snipped dried apricots
¼	cup orange marmalade

In medium saucepan combine water and sugar. Bring to a boil, stirring to dissolve sugar. Boil rapidly for 5 minutes. Add cranberries to sugar mixture, heat to just boiling, and reduce heat. Boil gently over medium heat for 3 to 4 minutes or until most of the cranberries' skins pop, stirring constantly. Stir in apricots and marmalade. Remove from heat. Serve warm or cold. Add a small amount of water, if necessary, to reach desired consistency.

Charlotte LaCrosse
Rockland, Maine

Tester's Note: Excellent combination of fruit flavors. Could be served with scones or English muffins for breakfast or tea.

cranberry Juice cooler

"Good for all, including sick, elderly and infants."

Preparation Time: 1 minute

1 serving

8   ounces cranberry juice
1   scoop lemon sherbet

Put scoop of sherbet in glass of cranberry juice and serve.

Dr. Philip Thompson
Portland, Maine

Summer Nectar

Preparation Time: 5 minutes

2 quarts

1   46-ounce jar apricot juice
1   banana
2   cups plain, nonfat yogurt
½   cup honey
     Strawberries, 6 or more

Put all ingredients in a blender and mix. Store up to a week in the refrigerator. After storing, stir before using.

Connie Thurston
Bethel, Maine

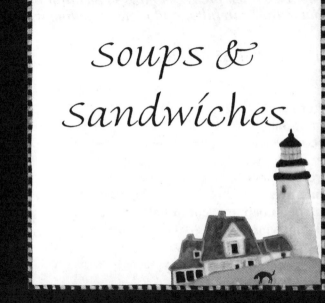

Soups & Sandwiches

Gazpacho

"This is an excellent soup for hot summer days. It is also a good way to use up the garden produce that is so plentiful then. It can be frozen, but defrost carefully. Add more seasoning if you like it spicier."

Preparation Time: 30 to 35 minutes

4 to 6 servings

3   cloves garlic
1   medium onion
1   small beet, peeled
1   medium cucumber
1   large green pepper
3   large tomatoes
2   small jalapeño peppers, cut in half and seeded
¼   cup red wine vinegar
¼   cup olive oil
¾   cup tomato juice
    Cumin to taste (optional)
4   drops Tabasco sauce
    Sour cream, cucumber slices, edible flowers or chopped
      parsley as garnish

In food processor, chop garlic and onion until fine. Add beet, cucumber, green pepper, tomatoes, jalapeño peppers, vinegar and olive oil. Chop until mixture is soup consistency. Add tomato juice, cumin and Tabasco sauce. Serve chilled and garnished with sour cream, cucumber slices, edible flowers (nasturtiums are colorful) or chopped parsley.

Lyn Donahue
Cumberland, Maine

Caution: Be careful seeding the jalapeño peppers (I wear gloves). Be sure to avoid touching eyes or mouth until hands are thoroughly washed with soap.

Spanish Summer Soup

Preparation Time: 15 minutes

6 servings

½   cucumber
½   onion, red or white
½   avocado, peeled
½   teaspoon crumbled oregano
3   tablespoons olive oil
2   tablespoons wine vinegar
4   cups canned tomato juice
    Ice cubes
2   limes, cut into wedges

Cut off a few slices of cucumber and onion to use as garnish. Chop remainder in small pieces. Slice or chop avocado. Put cucumber, onion, avocado, oregano, oil and vinegar in serving bowl (or blender, if you would like a smoother consistency). Pour in tomato juice and chill. Ladle into bowls and top with reserved cucumber and onion slices, adding 2 or 3 ice cubes to each bowl. Serve with lime wedges.

Phyllis Kindt
Santa Rosa, California

Tester's Note: While this quick and easy soup is intended to be served cold, it is also very good served hot. Spicy vegetable juice can substitute for the tomato juice with excellent results.

Broccoli Yogurt Soup

Preparation Time: 20 minutes

Cooking Time: 22 minutes

6 to 8 servings

1½ pounds broccoli
1   cup diced onion
1   tablespoon butter or margarine
5   cups chicken stock
½   teaspoon curry
½   teaspoon nutmeg
     Salt (optional)
     Pepper to taste
2   cups plain, non-fat yogurt

Rinse broccoli and cut into 1-inch chunks. In skillet sauté onions in butter/margarine until transparent. In large saucepan bring broth to a boil. Add broccoli, reduce heat, cover and simmer for 6 to 7 minutes until broccoli is slightly soft. Add onion and curry. Cook 10 to 15 minutes more. Remove from heat. Purée mixture in blender or food processor. Return to heat and add nutmeg, optional salt, pepper and yogurt. Heat to just under a boil.

Susan Grondin
Raymond, Maine

Tester's Note: The yogurt can be omitted for a dairy-free version. The taste is still excellent and it makes 4 ample servings.

Broccoli Cheese Soup

*"This recipe has passed through the hands of many friends.
It is delicious served the next day - even cold!"*

Preparation Time: 20 minutes

10 to 12 servings

2	tablespoons oil
¾	cup chopped onion
6	cups water
6	chicken bouillon cubes
4	cups flat noodles
1	teaspoon salt
1	10-ounce package frozen, chopped broccoli
⅛	teaspoon garlic powder
6	cups milk
1	pound processed cheese loaf, cut in chunks
	Dash of pepper

In large saucepan, heat oil. Add onions and sauté for 3 minutes.
Add water and bouillon cubes and bring to a boil. Add noodles
and salt and cook for 3 minutes. Stir in broccoli and garlic and
cook for 4 minutes. Turn down heat and stir in milk, cheese and
pepper. Be careful not to scald milk, but make sure cheese is
thoroughly melted. Ladle into soup bowls.

Bibi Thompson
South Portland, Maine

**Tester's Note: You can easily turn this soup into an excellent
casserole by reducing the milk and substituting cheddar cheese
for the processed cheese.**

Zucchini Apple Soup

There is an old joke in New England about keeping one's car locked when parked during August/September lest one return to the car to find it filled with zucchini. Having this recipe just may make some folks hesitate to lock their cars.....

Preparation Time: 30 minutes

Cooking Time: 30 minutes

6 servings

1   medium onion, chopped
1   cooking apple, peeled, cored and chopped
2   tablespoons butter, melted
4   cups chicken broth
3   cups unpeeled, diced zucchini (about 3 medium-sized
      zucchini)
1¼ cups whipping cream
¼   teaspoon pepper

Sauté onion and apple in butter in a Dutch oven until tender. Add broth and zucchini; bring to a boil. Cover, reduce heat and simmer 30 minutes or until zucchini is tender. Spoon mixture into the container of an electric blender and process until smooth. Return zucchini mixture to Dutch oven; stir in cream and pepper. Cook over low heat, stirring constantly, until well heated.

The Waterford Inne (Barbara Vanderzanden)
Waterford, Maine

Tester's Note: This soup is delicious served cold as well as hot.

Savory Carrot Soup

Preparation Time: 25 minutes

Cooking Time: 30 minutes

4 servings

	Extra virgin olive oil
1	pound carrots, diced
1	large potato, diced
1	medium onion, peeled and chopped
1	teaspoon chervil
3	cups vegetable stock (broth)
	Juice from 1 orange
	Salt and pepper
	Chopped green part of a scallion to garnish

Heat oil in large saucepan over medium heat. Add carrots, potato, onion and chervil. Toss and cook gently for 5 minutes. Don't let it brown. Add vegetable stock, lower heat, partially cover and simmer 30 minutes, or until vegetables are tender. Allow soup to cool slightly. Purée everything in blender. Add orange juice and seasonings, to taste. Garnish with scallions.

Vera Berv
Scarborough, Maine

Was okay, but didn't have chervil and have scallions, which would have made it sharper — May '11

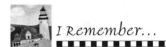

Butternut Squash Soup with Beet Drizzle

Preparation Time: 1 hour

6 to 8 servings

1	medium onion, roughly chopped
2	stalks celery, roughly chopped
2	carrots, roughly chopped
1	pound butternut squash, peeled, seeded and roughly chopped
2	bay leaves
3	cups chicken stock
	Salt and pepper to taste
1	large beet, peeled and roughly chopped
⅛	teaspoon grated nutmeg

Put onion, celery, carrots and squash in a large stock pot. Add chicken stock, bay leaves, salt and pepper. Cook over medium heat until all vegetables are soft, approximately 35 to 45 minutes. Meanwhile, boil beet in 1 quart of water until soft. (Add more water if it evaporates.) Drain. Purée beet in blender. Add nutmeg, salt, pepper and enough water for desired consistency - not too runny, not too thick. Place beet mixture in small sauce pan, ready to reheat. When vegetable mixture is done, remove bay leaves, add salt and pepper and purée in batches in blender. (Do not fill blender more than half full. Be careful not to get burned.) Ladle soup into warmed soup bowls and garnish with reheated beet drizzle.

Hugo's Portland Bistro (David Smith, Executive Chef)
Portland, Maine

Note: Both components of this recipe may be made two days in advance if you are having a dinner party and want to do some preparation ahead. Gently reheat soup and beet drizzle, separately, over low heat.

Spiced Butternut Squash Soup

Preparation Time: 15 minutes

6 to 8 servings

Cooking Time: 1 hour 40 minutes

2   medium-sized butternut squash (about 3 pounds altogether)
1   tablespoon fresh ginger, minced (see directions)
1   tablespoon canola oil
1   teaspoon whole black or brown mustard seeds
1   medium yellow or white onion, finely diced or chopped
2   (or more) cups of water or stock
    Sea salt (found at whole food markets), to taste
    Lemon juice to taste
    Dairy or soy yogurt or sour cream to garnish (optional)
2-4 tablespoons chopped fresh cilantro or parsley to garnish

Preheat oven to 375°. Bake squash by placing them on a rack in oven for 1 to 1½ hours until they can be pierced with a toothpick. Remove skin and seeds. Chop flesh and measure 3 cups for soup. (Reserve remaining squash for another use.) Mince fresh ginger by cutting a circular piece about ¼ to ½-inch thick. Lay the flat side of a chopping knife on top of the slice and pound the ginger once...that brings out the flavor...now finely mince the ginger. Heat oil in large saucepan or skillet over medium heat. Add mustard seeds and sauté for a few seconds, or until they begin to crackle and pop. Add ginger, sauté for 15 seconds; add onion, stir well and sauté until it begins to brown, stirring occasionally. While onion is cooking, combine squash and 2 cups of water or stock in a blender or food processor. Purée until smooth, adding enough liquid to get a thick soup consistency. Add squash purée to saucepan or skillet, stir well, add salt to taste and allow to simmer for 5 to 10 minutes. Stir in lemon juice to taste. Serve each bowl of soup garnished with optional yogurt and chopped fresh cilantro.

Vera Berv
Scarborough, Maine

Note: For variety you can substitute plain, non-fat yogurt for one or more cups of the water/stock. This will give a tangier taste. Adjust the liquid and seasonings to suit yourself.

Curried Roasted Squash and Pear Soup

Preparation Time: 30 minutes

Cooking Time: 1 hour

8 cups

1	butternut squash (1½ pounds), peeled, seeded and cut into ¾-inch cubes
6	ripe, but firm, Bartlett pears, peeled, cored and cut into ¾-inch cubes
2	tablespoons olive oil, divided
1	teaspoon honey or brown rice syrup (available at whole foods markets)
	Sea salt and freshly ground black pepper to taste
½	cup water
⅓	cup finely chopped shallots
1	tablespoon packed dark brown sugar
1	2½-inch cinnamon stick
2	teaspoons curry powder
½	teaspoon ground cardamom
¼	teaspoon ground coriander
6	cups reduced-sodium chicken broth, defatted
2	tablespoons slivered fresh mint or cilantro leaves to garnish

Preheat oven to 400°. On large baking sheet with sides, toss squash and pears with 1 tablespoon oil and the honey/syrup. Season with salt and pepper. Drizzle with water. Roast squash and pears for 30 to 40 minutes or until both are tender. (Add a little more water, if necessary, to prevent burning.) Remove any pears that are done before squash. Measure 1 cup pears and cut each cube in half; set aside. In food processor or blender, purée squash and remaining pears until smooth. (Add a little chicken broth, if necessary.) Set aside. In a soup pot, heat remaining tablespoon oil over medium heat. Add shallots and cook, stirring, until softened, but not browned, 3 to 5 minutes. Add brown sugar, cinnamon stick, curry powder, cardamom and coriander. Stir for 2 minutes more. Add reserved squash-pear purée and chicken broth. Bring to a simmer. Reduce heat to low and simmer, stirring occasionally, for 25 to 30 minutes. Season with salt and pepper. Discard cinnamon stick. Add reserved pears and simmer until heated through. Ladle into warmed soup bowls and garnish with mint or cilantro. Serve immediately.

Vera Berv
Scarborough, Maine

Pumpkin Apple Soup

Four generations of our Irish family have used this simple and inexpensive soup at Thanksgiving as a dinner starter to get everyone to the table. But I think the tradition really started because the turkey, etc., needed to be stretched, given the average annual gathering includes 25+ people!!

Preparation Time: 30 minutes

8 cups

1-2 tablespoons butter
1   medium onion, chopped (½ cup)
1   clove garlic, minced
3   cups fresh or canned chicken stock
1   16-ounce can pumpkin
1   tablespoon sugar
¼   teaspoon ground cinnamon
2   tart apples (like Granny Smith), coarsely chopped
1   cup whipping cream or evaporated milk
     Salt and freshly ground black pepper to taste
     Parsley or watercress sprigs to garnish

Melt butter in heavy, large saucepan or soup pot. Add onion and garlic and cook over medium heat until tender but not brown (3 to 4 minutes). Stir in broth, pumpkin, sugar and cinnamon. Add the apples. Heat mixture until boiling. Cover, reduce heat and simmer 10 minutes. Add cream/evaporated milk. Purée a portion at a time using blender or food processor. Return all to saucepan. Heat through. Season to taste with salt and pepper. Garnish with parsley or watercress sprigs.

Pat Lambrew
Scarborough, Maine

Parsnip Soup with Butternut Squash and Roasted Red Pepper

"I really enjoy making soups as well as eating them. I really like to use whatever is local and in season to do this. This soup is a good fall or spring soup for these reasons. But you can get parsnips pretty much all year long at the grocery store."

Preparation Time: 45 to 60 minutes

6 to 8 servings

4	tablespoons butter
6	large parsnips, peeled and coarsely chopped
1	large onion, diced
3	cloves garlic, peeled and smashed
½	teaspoon fresh chopped rosemary
3	quarts vegetable or chicken stock
1	cup peeled and finely-diced butternut squash
1	medium to small red pepper, finely diced
2	tablespoons olive oil
4	cups heavy cream
	Salt and pepper to taste

Preheat broiler. In heavy stock pot, melt butter and heat until it becomes nutty brown. Add parsnips, onion and garlic and sauté until garlic becomes slightly caramelized. Add rosemary and enough stock to cover by ½-inch and bring to boil. Then reduce to a fast simmer. While mixture simmers, toss squash and red pepper separately, each with a tablespoon of olive oil. Place on separate sheet pans and broil until they start to caramelize. Pull out and stir around on the pans. Return to oven to caramelize the other side. Remove when this is done and cool. When parsnip mixture has cooked enough to become soft, add cream and mash with a potato masher. (For a smoother consistency, use a blender.) If mixture is too thick, add any remaining stock, or add water, to achieve desired consistency. Texture and thickness is an individual thing. I prefer mine done differently each time, depending on my mood. Put soup back on stove, bring to a simmer and continue simmering over low heat for 5 minutes. Add squash and pepper. Reheat, season and serve.

Fore Street Restaurant (Sous Chef: Esau Crosby II)
Portland, Maine

Tester's Note: It is possible to substitute yogurt for the heavy cream with excellent results. If you like spicy food, add a little hot sauce. The soup is wonderful hot or cold!

Spring Pea Soup

Preparation Time: 30 minutes

8 servings

2   stalks celery, diced
1   small white onion, diced
¾   stick butter
4   cups chicken stock
1   pound shelled fresh peas
1   cup heavy cream
    Salt and pepper to taste
2   tablespoons mint, finely chopped, as garnish

In large saucepan, soften celery and onion in butter over low heat. Add chicken stock and bring to a boil over high heat. When stock is boiling, add shelled peas. Bring back to a boil. Remove from heat and strain, reserving liquid. (Also, reserve enough peas to garnish 8 servings.) In blender or food processor, process the vegetable mixture with just enough liquid to purée. Return to clean pot. Repeat process, if necessary, until all vegetables are puréed. Some liquid may remain. Use it to thin the purée if it is too thick. Strain mixture through a strainer and push some solids through. Add cream and bring to a simmer. Season with salt and pepper. Garnish with mint and reserved peas.

Harraseeket Inn
Freeport, Maine

Cream of Fiddlehead Soup

"The month of May in Maine brings 'Fiddleheads', a true delicacy found in stores and markets during the season. But the most fun is looking for the little ostrich ferns and gathering them yourself. The fiddlehead is covered with a brown, onion-skin-type covering, which helps to identify it. Be sure to remove this covering (markets usually do this). To further clean, tap or shake each fiddlehead gently to get rid of any remaining brown flecks. Then wash well and they are ready for steaming, sautéing or to use in this delicious soup."

Preparation Time: 30 minutes

Cooking Time: 30 minutes

10 to 12 servings

⅓ cup flour
½ cup butter (1 stick) or equivalent volume vegetable oil
1 large onion, diced
1 pound fresh fiddleheads, cleaned
1-2 cups water
3 16-ounce cans chicken stock
   Salt and pepper to taste
1 heaping tablespoon sugar
1 pint cream (or half-and-half or whole milk)
   Plain yogurt or sour cream to garnish
   Chopped parsley, chives or chive flowers to garnish

In a large saucepan, over medium-high heat, make a roux with flour and butter, stirring constantly for 1 to 2 minutes (do not brown). Add onion and cook, continuing to stir, until onions are wilted, but not browned. Add fiddleheads and water. Increase heat to high, bring to a boil; then cover and remove from heat. When lukewarm to cool, using a plastic spatula, scrape pan contents into a food processor and finely purée. Return to saucepan and rinse processor with a small amount of water to capture all purée. Add chicken stock and bring to a boil, stirring frequently; then reduce heat to simmer. Add salt, pepper and sugar. Simmer for 20 minutes; add cream, half-and-half, or milk. Again, bring to a simmer for 10 to 15 minutes. Remove from heat, let sit for 15 to

20 minutes and serve. You might save a few fiddleheads before puréeing to lay onto a tablespoon of yogurt or sour cream as a garnish. Alternatively, garnish with chopped parsley or chives; or, for vibrant color, top each serving with chive flowers, which share the season with fiddleheads.

Brian M. Dorsk
Cape Elizabeth, Maine

Note: Amount of flour can be adjusted to achieve desired consistency. Choices of butter versus vegetable oil and cream versus half-and-half or milk depend on the needs or tolerance of your coronary arteries!

Easy Peasy Soup

"Here is an infallible 'quickie' recipe which has stood me in good stead over the years as a single, working mother living in London and in need of a good wife! Now a wide-eyed tourist in Maine for a couple of years, it still features regularly on my table."

Preparation Time: 8 minutes

6 to 8 servings as a first course

3　15-ounce cans petite sweet peas
1　7-ounce container basil pesto
1　cup light cream
1　large chicken bouillon cube
　　Fresh basil leaves as garnish

In food processor, blend 2 cans of undrained peas with pesto and bouillon cube for about 3 minutes. Pour into large saucepan, add last can of undrained peas and cream, reserving a little cream for garnish, and mix together. Heat and serve, drizzling each serving with remaining cream and topping with a basil leaf or two.

Melody MacDonald
Scarborough, Maine

Scallion Soup

"I discovered this while reading a magazine - waiting for lunch to arrive in a local restaurant. The recipe called for squid as an ingredient, but it got a more enthusiastic reception without it. Everybody loves this soup!"

Preparation Time: 30 minutes

Cooking Time: 50 to 55 minutes

6 or more servings

3	tablespoons butter
1	pound scallions, sliced
¼	cup flour
6	cups warm vegetable or chicken broth
	Salt and pepper
1	tablespoon olive oil
1	shallot (or onion), chopped
1	bunch Swiss chard (not red), coarse middle ribs removed, leaves chopped
½	cup peas

In sauce pan, heat butter and add scallions. Sauté until tender. Stir in flour and cook for 1 minute. Pour in warm broth, slowly, whisking as you pour. Season with salt and pepper. Cover and simmer for 50 minutes. 10 minutes before scallion mixture is done, in large sauce pan, heat olive oil with shallot. Add Swiss chard and peas. Simmer 6 to 7 minutes. Purée scallion mixture in a blender . When chard and peas are done, stir in scallion purée and serve.

Vera Berv
Scarborough, Maine

carol's comfort chicken soup

"There was no holiday at my family's house without chicken soup. All the warmth of the gatherings was enriched by this ritual of sipping together."

Preparation Time: 2½ hours

8 quarts

1   3- to 4-pound fowl, pullet or whole chicken
2   whole chicken breasts
2   parsnips, peeled and chunked
4   stalks celery, cut in big chunks
4   carrots, peeled and chunked
2-3 onions, peeled and chunked
    Salt and pepper to taste
1   12-ounce package matzoh meal or 1 16-ounce package egg
    noodles, cooked

Place chicken in 6 to 8-quart soup pot. Cover with water (approximately 3 quarts), bring to boil and simmer 20 minutes. Skim "debris" off the top. Add the vegetables and simmer 1½ hours. Remove chicken. Remove bones and cut up meat (saving some for sandwiches). Remove vegetables and place in a blender to purée. Add the puréed vegetables to the broth in the soup pot. Add chicken. You may now add the matzoh balls you have prepared following the directions on the matzoh meal package, or you may add the cooked egg noodles to the broth.

Carol Rabinovitz
Cumberland Foreside, Maine

Note: Adding the puréed vegetables is a good way to "trick" the kids into eating their vegetables!

Roasted Plum Tomato and Salmon Soup

"This recipe was given to me by one of the best cooks I know, my friend, Alix. Friends since early childhood, we have shared a great deal together, including both of our mothers' struggles with Alzheimer's disease."

Preparation Time: 1 hour

6 to 8 servings

4	pounds ripe plum tomatoes, halved lengthwise
3	tablespoons butter
1	red onion, chopped
2	large stalks celery, thinly sliced
2	carrots, shredded
3	cloves garlic, chopped
8	cups chicken stock
2	tablespoons chopped fresh parsley
1	tablespoon chopped fresh tarragon
1	cup medium barley
	Salt and pepper to taste
1	tablespoon lemon juice
1	cup dry white wine
2	pounds skinless salmon, cut in 1-inch chunks
	Lite sour cream and chopped scallions to garnish

Preheat broiler. Line baking pan with aluminum foil. Place tomato halves, skin side up, on baking sheet. Roast about 6 inches from heat until tomato skins are charred and blackened, about 8 to 10 minutes. Remove from oven and, when cool enough to handle, slip off skins and gently squeeze to dislodge the seeds. Coarsely chop tomatoes and set aside. Melt butter in a 4-quart Dutch oven. Add onion, celery, carrots and garlic and cook over medium heat until the vegetables begin to wilt, about 5 minutes. Stir in roasted tomatoes. Add chicken stock. Simmer uncovered for 15 minutes. Add parsley, tarragon and barley. Cover and cook for an additional 20 to 25 minutes until the barley is tender. Season to taste with salt and pepper; add lemon juice, wine and salmon. Simmer 5 to 8 minutes, or until the fish flakes easily with a fork.

Add a dollop of sour cream and sprinkle with scallions. Serve immediately.

Carolyn Cooper McGoldrick
Cape Elizabeth, Maine

chicken and Rice Soup

Preparation Time: 45 minutes

12 to 16 servings

6   cups water
6-8 chicken bouillon cubes
5   carrots, chopped
1   cup chopped celery
1   large onion, chopped
    Salt and pepper to taste
    Seasonings to taste
1   14½-ounce can tomatoes
3-4 pound chicken, cooked, skin and bones removed, cut-up
1   cup rice, uncooked

In a 5-quart soup pot, heat water to boiling. Add bouillon cubes, carrots, celery, onion and seasonings. Bring back to a boil, lower heat and add undrained tomatoes. Simmer 30 minutes. Add chicken and rice. Simmer another 20 minutes. (Can use crock pot and simmer all day. Add rice for the last 20 minutes.)

Joyce Kidney, Caregiver
Brewer, Maine

Shrimp Bisque

Preparation Time: 60 minutes

2 quarts

¼   carrot, small dice
½   onion, small dice
¼   celery stalk, small dice
½   small garlic clove, minced
1½ tablespoons butter
½   pound shrimp, peeled (divided)
1   quart chicken stock (homemade or from Stone Soup)
½   head cauliflower, small dice
    Dash of cayenne
    White pepper to taste
⅛   teaspoon black pepper
½   cup cream
    Chopped parsley to garnish

In large soup pot sauté first 4 ingredients in butter until translucent. Add ½ the shrimp and sauté until done (2 to 3 minutes). Add chicken stock, cauliflower, and seasonings and simmer until cauliflower is cooked. Purée the mixture in blender, return to pot and add the remaining shrimp. Cook for 3 minutes. Pour cream in small bowl. Add some warm soup to the cold cream to "temper" before adding cream to the hot soup. Garnish each bowl with chopped parsley.

Stone Soup (Chefs: Chris Cole and Caite Maynard)
Portland, Maine

Grandfather Gould's Fish Chowder

"Grandfather Gould and Uncle Oliver used this recipe on their fishing trips in the 1890's. They would take potatoes, onions and 'salt pork' with them and stop in at farmhouses to buy cream and butter for their chowder. Tastes even better the second day!"

Preparation Time: 40 minutes

Cooking Time: 15 to 20 minutes

8 to 10 servings

6	strips bacon, minced
2	tablespoons butter
2	large onions, diced
6	medium potatoes, cubed
1½-2	pounds fresh haddock
6	cups water
	Salt and pepper
1	quart heavy cream, light cream or milk (as you prefer)

Place bacon in 6-quart pot and sauté over medium heat until cooked. Add butter and onion and cook until onions are transparent. Place potatoes on onion mixture. Add enough water to cover potatoes. Place fish on top of potatoes. Bring to a boil, reduce heat, cover and simmer for about 15 to 20 minutes or until the potatoes are soft, but not overcooked. Fish should flake and break up easily. Remove from heat. Stir and add salt and pepper to taste. Warm cream, add to mixture and stir. Ladle into soup bowls.

Ann Noyes
Yarmouth, Maine

Ann's Seafood Chowder

"For many years a group of neighbors have celebrated Christmas Eve with an early potluck supper at our home. The menu itself has become a tradition with this seafood chowder holding a place of honor. It is just one of my own family's favorites made by my friend Ann, an outstanding cook and loving daughter of Marie, another person with Alzheimer's."

Preparation Time: 20 to 25 minutes

8 servings

4   cups unpeeled, diced, red potatoes
¼   cup chopped onion
2   6½-ounce cans chopped clams
1   stick butter
3-4   tablespoons flour
1   quart half-and-half
½   pound crabmeat
½   pound uncooked shrimp, peeled
½   pound scallops
½   pound haddock or cod
1½   teaspoons salt
½   teaspoon pepper
½   teaspoon sugar
       Dill, fresh or dried, to taste

Place potatoes and onion in top of double boiler. Drain juice from clams over vegetables with enough added water to cover. Simmer until potatoes are just tender. While vegetables cook, melt butter in saucepan. Add flour and blend. Cook 1 to 2 minutes. Add half-and-half and cook, stirring, until smooth and thick. Add to vegetables along with all the seafood. Cook until fish is flaky. Add salt, pepper, sugar and a dash of dill. Serve immediately.

Carolyn Cooper McGoldrick
Cape Elizabeth, Maine

Baked Fish Chowder

"Smells divine while cooking! Lifted, with modification, from a long-time co-worker's recipe file."

Preparation Time: 15 minutes

Baking Time: 1 hour

4 to 6 servings

1	onion, sliced
1	potato, sliced
	Minced garlic to taste
1	teaspoon dill
2	tablespoons butter
1	cup clam juice or water, boiling
1	pound haddock or salmon fillet
1	cup cream or rich milk, warmed

Layer first 7 ingredients in casserole with cover, fish on top. Cover and bake for 60 minutes. Add cream or milk, stir gently and serve.

Connie Korda
Falmouth, Maine

Suggestion: If using salmon in place of haddock, place fillet on top with skin side up. Upon completion of baking, skin peels off easily. So easy and delicious, you'll never make it another way!

Hearty Minestrone

"This recipe came from a friend, "Aunt Rita" Brunelleschi, in Florence in 1950. My husband had met her during World War II when she was working with the Red Cross. Our children call this recipe 100 Vegetable Soup. Feel free to vary vegetables and to add broccoli, cabbage, zucchini or left-overs."

Preparation Time: 30 minutes

Cooking Time: 3 to 4 hours

8 to 10 hearty servings

1	pound stew meat, cut small
2	onions, chopped
2	stalks celery, chopped
2	potatoes, diced
2	cloves garlic, minced
3	tablespoons chopped parsley
1	16-ounce can kidney beans
1	32-ounce can Italian tomatoes
	Water (optional), up to 2-quarts to achieve desired consistency
1	8-ounce can corn
1	8-ounce can peas
1	8-ounce can green beans
2	teaspoons salt, or to taste
½	teaspoon pepper
1	teaspoon oregano
1½	cups pasta, cooked

Put all ingredients, except pasta, in crock pot or large kettle. Simmer slowly 3 to 4 hours. Add water from time to time as necessary. Adjust seasonings and add pasta. Serve with French or Italian bread as a main course.

Polly Wright
Mendon, Vermont

Tester's Note: This wonderful soup can also be made with no meat, using chicken stock in place of water. If you do use meat, you might consider browning it first in a little oil or butter. Fresh or frozen vegetables can replace the canned ones, if you prefer.

Spicy African Rice and Peanut Soup

Preparation Time: 40 minutes

12 to 15 servings

1	tablespoon vegetable oil
1	large onion, chopped
1	medium sweet potato, peeled and diced
2	cloves garlic, minced
8	cups chicken broth
1	teaspoon dried thyme leaves
½	teaspoon ground cumin
1	cup uncooked long grain rice
2	cups thick and chunky salsa
1	19-ounce can garbanzo beans (chickpeas), drained and rinsed
1	cup diced unpeeled zucchini
⅔	cup creamy peanut butter (low-fat variety is fine)

In large pot, heat oil and sauté onions, sweet potato and garlic, stirring occasionally until onion is soft, about 5 minutes. Add chicken broth, thyme, cumin and rice. Bring to a boil, reduce heat and simmer, covered, until rice is cooked and vegetables are tender, about 18 to 20 minutes. Add salsa, beans and zucchini; cook until zucchini is tender, about 10 minutes. Add peanut butter and stir until completely combined.

Constance Turcotte
Cape Elizabeth, Maine

Pasta e Fagioli

Preparation Time: 30 minutes

Cooking Time: 30 minutes

12 to 15 servings

1	pound pasta (small or medium shells, or your choice)
1	cup minced prosciutto
½	cup minced pancetta
1	carrot, diced
½	red onion, diced
3	stalks celery, diced
3½	cups white wine
1	32-ounce can plum tomatoes
2	bay leaves
½	teaspoon oregano
5	8-ounce cans cannellini beans
	Salt and pepper to taste

Cook pasta as directed on package, drain, and set aside. In soup pot brown prosciutto and pancetta. Add carrot, onion, and celery and brown. Add white wine and bring to a boil. Add tomatoes, bay leaves, oregano, and beans. Bring to a boil again; turn heat down, cover and simmer for 30 minutes, stirring occasionally. Add salt and pepper to taste. Stir in cooked pasta and serve.

Casa Napoli Ristorante (Daniel Call, Executive Chef)
Falmouth, Maine

Irish Stew

"This stew with biscuits was a warm, nurturing meal served by Mom on cold rainy days and in winter. I have added a bay leaf and changed from the use of oil to nonstick cooking spray."

Preparation Time: 30 minutes

Cooking Time: 2½ hours

4 to 6 servings

1½ pounds stew beef
    Non-stick cooking spray
3-4 potatoes, cubed
1   pound carrots, sliced
4-5 celery stalks, sliced
1   medium onion, sliced
    Salt and pepper to taste
1   large bay leaf
    Beef bouillon cubes (optional)

Brown stew beef in large pot sprayed with nonstick cooking spray. Cover beef with water after browning and simmer, covered, 2 hours. Watch water level and add more, if necessary. Add vegetables to stew. Add more water to cover. Bring to a boil, reduce heat, cover and simmer for another ½ hour, adding bay leaf for the last 20 minutes. Add salt and pepper to taste. Add optional bouillon cubes for the last 10 minutes. Add water to make it as thin or thick as you like. Broth will be clear.

Elizabeth McLeod
South Portland, Maine

Beef and Apple Stew

Preparation Time: 45 minutes

Cooking Time: 2 hours

8 servings

⅓   cup flour
1   teaspoon salt
¼   teaspoon pepper
½   teaspoon paprika
2   pounds stew beef, cut in 1½-inch cubes
3   tablespoons cooking oil
1   large onion, cut in quarters
2   cups apple juice
2   medium apples
1   cup sliced celery
3   large carrots, peeled and sliced
1   small turnip, peeled and cut in ½-inch sticks
1   bay leaf
¼   teaspoon oregano
     Salt and pepper to taste

Combine flour, salt, pepper, and paprika in a bag. Add meat cubes
and shake to coat. Heat oil in heavy, large saucepan or soup pot;
add meat and brown. Add onions and apple juice; bring to a boil.
Turn down heat, cover, and simmer for 1 hour. Peel, core, and
slice apples. Add to stew with celery, carrots, turnip and
remaining seasonings. Cover and simmer 1 hour. Serve with
mashed potatoes or as a stew.

Churchill Caterers and Event Planners
Portland, Maine

No Peek Stew

Preparation Time: 10 minutes

Baking Time: 3 hours

4 to 6 servings

2 pounds boneless beef stew meat, cut into 1½-inch cubes
1 10¾-ounce can condensed cream soup (mushroom or chicken)
1 envelope onion soup mix
1 cup water
6-8 ounces wide noodles
2 tablespoons butter
  Chopped parsley as garnish (optional)

Preheat oven to 350°. In 3-quart casserole, combine stew meat, canned soup, onion soup mix and water. Mix well. Cover and bake for 3 hours. When nearly done, prepare noodles according to package directions. Drain and add butter. To serve, spoon stew on top of noodles. Garnish with parsley, if desired.

Gloria C. Daigle
Madawaska, Maine

MaMere's Beef Stew

"Everyone, of all generations, loved this plain meat and potato dish. No one ever tried to change it or add a spice or substitute ingredients. It's always been a comfort food for bad weather nights or tummy ache days."

Preparation Time: 20 minutes

6 servings

½	pound lean ground beef
1	large onion, chopped
1½-2	quarts water
	Salt and pepper to taste
3	potatoes, cut up
2	tablespoons flour

In a large saucepan cook together ground beef, onion, water, salt and pepper until meat is done. Add potatoes and cook until tender. Stir flour into a little cold water, then add mixture to the soup. Stir until blended and thickened.

Priscilla Verrier
Biddeford, Maine

carrot Sandwich Spread

"Great for large gatherings. Used several times for Memory Walk. People can't believe it's carrots!"

Preparation Time: ½ hour

6 cups

6	medium carrots
¼	small onion, chopped
½	medium green pepper, chopped
1	tablespoon pimiento, chopped
½	cup chopped walnuts
½-1	cup mayonnaise or salad dressing
1	large Pullman loaf of bread

Chop carrots in food processor until fine. Drain off any liquid, if necessary. Put in bowl and add onion, green pepper, pimiento, walnuts and mayonnaise or salad dressing until mixture is moist and spreadable. Make sandwiches using the entire loaf of bread.

Marilyn Paige
Scarborough, Maine

Tester's Note: Can also be used as an appetizer spread on rounds of French bread or party rye.

Barbara's Mediterranean Loaf

"This recipe comes from a fabulous Virginia chef (whose father was a doctor and who delivered my husband!). We ate this bread on a porch in spring in Virginia surrounded by beautiful blooming azaleas."

Preparation Time: 30 minutes

4 to 6 servings

1   long loaf French or Italian bread
1½ cups chopped tomatoes
½   cup thinly sliced scallions
⅓   cup pimiento-stuffed green olives, chopped
⅓   cup Greek black olives, pitted and chopped
½   cup minced fresh parsley
1   tablespoon capers
1   tablespoon minced fresh basil (or 1 teaspoon dried)
2-3 tablespoons olive oil
     Salt and pepper to taste

Cut the ends off bread and cut bread into 2 or 3 sections. Using a long, thin knife, hollow out bread, reserving crumbs. Leave shell about ½-inch thick. Pulverize (in food processor) or tear reserved crumbs and mix with remaining ingredients. (Can all be done in food processor using pulse.) Pack stuffing in bread shells and wrap tightly in foil. Chill for at least 8 hours or overnight. Slice with serrated knife and serve.

Hillary Dorsk
Cape Elizabeth, Maine

Note: Serve for lunch or as an appetizer. Great on picnics with cheese, fruits, meats and/or shrimp on the side!

cheese Dreams

"Quick and easy, Cheese Dreams were a spur-of-the-minute meal. We always had the fixings on hand. My parents had a Magic Chef stove with the broiler on top of the stove. In my own house here in Maine I have the fixings all the time."

Preparation Time: 15 minutes

4 servings

4	slices white bread
2	cups grated extra sharp cheddar cheese
1	teaspoon Worcestershire sauce
1	ripe tomato, sliced thin
8	bacon strips, cut in half

Preheat broiler. Lightly toast bread and place on broiler pan. In bowl combine cheese and Worcestershire sauce. Mix well and spoon on top of the 4 bread slices. Top each with tomato slices. Then top each with 4 pieces of bacon. Broil until bubbly, about 2 minutes.

Betty A. Small
Yarmouth, Maine

Quick Hot Sandwich

"Differently delicious and simple."

Preparation Time: 20 minutes

15 to 20 open-faced sandwiches

1   loaf French bread
½   stick butter
1   15-ounce can whole berry cranberry sauce
1   8-ounce block cheddar cheese

Preheat broiler. Slice bread. Toast lightly on both sides. Butter one side. Spread layer of cranberry sauce over butter and top with thin slice of cheddar cheese. Broil until cheese is bubbly (or heat in microwave oven).

Joan Hyde
Yarmouth, Maine

Humbugs

Preparation Time: 30 minutes

3 dozen

1   small onion
1   small green pepper
4   hard-boiled eggs
1   pound cooked ham
1   pound cheese
2   10¾-ounce cans tomato soup
18 English muffins, split and toasted

Preheat broiler to medium. Grind or finely chop first 5 ingredients. Mix with tomato soup. Place mixture on English muffins. Broil until cheese is melted and/or until muffins start to brown.

Donna Landry
Mexico, Maine

Quesadillas

"I serve this to my children, as a snack, with hot Mexican chocolate when they get home from school. It has now become a family tradition."

Preparation Time: 2 minutes

12 servings

12 8-inch tortillas (corn or flour)
4   cups shredded cheddar cheese
    Diced chicken (optional)
    Diced onion (optional)

Place a generous amount of cheese in center of tortilla and fold in half. Cook lightly in hot, ungreased skillet, turning once or twice until cheese is melted.

Hilde H. Royer
Falmouth, Maine

Portobello Sandwich

Preparation Time: 10 minutes

2 servings

2	small focaccia breads (or 1 large, cut in half)

3-4 ounces goat cheese
1   tablespoon olive oil, divided
1   portobello mushroom, sliced
1   tablespoon white wine
1   clove garlic, minced
     ⅛ teaspoon salt
     Pepper to taste
8   strips marinated red peppers
1   avocado, peeled and sliced

If focaccia is too thick, pull out soft middle of breads and use the shells. Spread goat cheese on 2 breads. Sauté portobello slices in ½ tablespoon oil. Layer slices on goat cheese. Mix together wine, garlic, remaining oil, salt and pepper. Dribble over mushrooms. Top with peppers and avocado. Heat in microwave oven.

Nan Delaney
Denver, Colorado

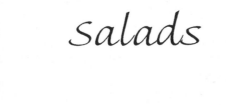

salads

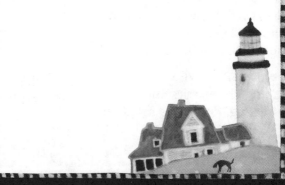

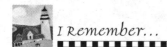

Speedy Salad Delight

"Wonderfully simple, quick and tasty"

Preparation Time: 10 minutes

10 to 14 servings

3   5-ounce packages spring salad greens (mixed)
1   16-ounce can pears (light syrup), drained, reserving
       ⅓ to ½ cup syrup
½-1 cup crumbled feta cheese
½-1 cup dried cranberries or raisins
½   cup chopped pecans
⅓-½ cup bottled Dijon honey mustard dressing

Place greens in salad bowl. Cut pears into small pieces and add with feta cheese, cranberries and nuts. Mix reserved pear syrup and Dijon dressing. Pour onto salad and toss.

Barbara Boucher
Denver, Colorado

Ruby's Cole Slaw

"This recipe was given to me by a friend I worked with at a shoe factory years ago. It keeps a long time if kept cold."

Preparation Time: ½ hour

8 to 10 servings

1	large head cabbage
2	carrots
1	onion
½	cup sugar
¾	cup vinegar
1	teaspoon celery seed
1	teaspoon mustard seed
½	teaspoon salt
¾	cup corn oil

Chop cabbage, carrot and onion, and mix together in large bowl. Mix all other ingredients and heat but don't boil. Cool. Pour over cabbage mixture and toss well.

Ruby Stambaugh
St. James, Missouri

Spinach Salad

Preparation Time: 30 minutes

6 to 8 servings

1	pound fresh spinach, washed, dried and torn into bite-sized pieces
6	hard-boiled eggs, coarsely chopped
6	slices bacon, cooked and crumbled

Salad Dressing

½	cup salad oil
¼	cup sugar
2	tablespoons red wine vinegar
1	teaspoon finely grated onion
½	teaspoon salt
¼	teaspoon dry mustard

Layer first 3 ingredients in a bowl and chill. Mix together salad dressing ingredients until thick and the sugar has dissolved. Chill. When ready to serve pour dressing on spinach mixture and toss.

Betsy Bracken Barrett
Scarborough, Maine

Spinach Apple Salad

Preparation Time: 20 minutes

6 servings

1   pound fresh spinach leaves, washed, dried and torn into bite-sized pieces
½   cup walnuts, coarsely chopped (toasted, if desired)
¼   pound cheddar cheese, cut into cubes
1   apple, skin left on, cut into cubes
6   slices bacon, cooked and cut into pieces

Dressing
⅓   cup cider vinegar
½   small onion, chopped
1   teaspoon salt, or to taste
1   teaspoon dry mustard
½-¾   cup sugar
1   cup vegetable oil
1½   tablespoons poppy seeds

Make dressing. In blender or food processor blend vinegar, onion, salt, mustard and sugar until smooth. With blender turned on, add oil in thin stream. Blend until smooth. Stir in poppy seeds. Refrigerate until ready to use. Combine salad ingredients in salad bowl. Pour on dressing to taste and toss.

Dot Cleveland
South Portland, Maine

Pear Walnut Salad

"This recipe came from a close friend who lives in Virginia. We visit back and forth a couple times a year. Meals are kept simple and we try and come up with new foods to share. We have enjoyed this one very much."

Preparation Time: 20 minutes

4 servings

4	cups torn lettuce
1	large (or 2 small) pears
¼	cup toasted walnuts
2	ounces blue cheese, crumbled
½	cup oil
3	tablespoons cider vinegar
¼	teaspoon salt
¼	teaspoon celery seed
3	tablespoons sugar

Put lettuce in bowl. Wash, core and slice or chop pears. Add pears to lettuce. Toast walnuts in 350° oven for 5 to 6 minutes. Combine remaining ingredients except blue cheese and mix well. Pour dressing over lettuce and pears and toss until just coated. (Save remaining dressing for another salad.) Add nuts and blue cheese. Toss and serve.

Dorothy G. Larkin
Cumberland Foreside, Maine

Mandarin Salad

"A winner! Dressing can be refrigerated for about 1 week. It should be brought to room temperature in order to use."

Preparation Time: ½ hour

4 to 6 servings

⅓ cup sliced almonds
1 large head romaine lettuce, torn into pieces
  Cucumbers, peeled and sliced, to taste
1 10-ounce can mandarin oranges, chilled and drained

Poppy Seed Dressing
1 tablespoon red onion
1 teaspoon dry mustard
1 teaspoon salt
1 teaspoon paprika
½ cup sugar
1 cup salad oil
¼ cup wine vinegar
1 tablespoon poppy seeds

Preheat oven to 350°. Place foil on baking sheet and spread out almonds evenly on foil. Bake until medium brown, 5 to 7 minutes. Set aside. Make dressing; add onion, dry mustard, salt, paprika, and sugar to bowl of food processor. Turn on food processor and alternate dripping oil and vinegar through feed tube. When thoroughly mixed, put dressing in jar, add poppy seeds and shake. Mix romaine, cucumbers and oranges; toss with dressing to taste. Add almonds and toss lightly.

Margaret Wilkis
South Portland, Maine

Broccoli Salad

"Delicious, nutritious, crunchy salad."

Preparation Time: 30 minutes

6 servings

1   cup mayonnaise
2   tablespoons vinegar
½   cup sugar
2-3 heads broccoli, chopped into bite size pieces
1   small red onion, diced
½   pound bacon, cooked and chopped
½   cup unsalted sunflower seeds
½   cup raisins

Mix mayonnaise, vinegar and sugar. Add to rest of salad and chill.

Charlene Ferguson
Yarmouth, Maine

Tester's Note: I really liked this. Great without the bacon also.

Marinated Vegetables

"Whenever I have made this I have used fresh vegetables and cooked them al dente."

Preparation Time: 15 minutes

1	cup corn oil
1	cup vinegar
⅓	cup sugar
4	teaspoons salt, or to taste
½	teaspoon pepper
2	15½-ounce cans kidney beans, drained
2	15-ounce cans baby carrots, drained
½	cup finely chopped onion
3	10-ounce packages broccoli

Mix first 5 ingredients. Pour over vegetables; cover and refrigerate overnight. Drain and arrange vegetables on platter.

Dawn Leavitt
Kezar Falls, Maine

Tester's Note: Can use any combination of vegetables.

Sorrel Salad

"Looking back I think that one of the things that really attracted me to Maine was the quality of the raw ingredients that I had in front of me to cook with. The variety is enormous. This is one of my favorite recipes utilizing local products."

Preparation Time: 15 minutes

2 servings

1   bunch sorrel (10 to 12 leaves), tough stems removed
6   stalks pencil asparagus, blanched and cut in half
4   tablespoons high quality olive oil (such as Nunez de Prado)
     Sea salt and course ground pepper to taste
     Fresh Parmesan cheese such as Reggiano, shaved from a
       block, to taste

Combine sorrel, asparagus and olive oil in a mixing bowl.
Season with salt, pepper and shaved Parmesan cheese.

Gabriel's
Portland, Maine

crunchy pea Salad

Preparation Time: 15 minutes

8 servings

1	10-ounce package frozen peas, thawed
1	8-ounce can water chestnuts, drained
1	cup thinly sliced celery
2	tablespoons sugar
½	teaspoon curry powder
½	cup sliced green onion
4	tablespoons lemon juice
1	teaspoon dill weed
½	teaspoon salt
¼	teaspoon pepper
¼	cup mayonnaise
¼	cup sour cream

Mix all ingredients except mayonnaise and sour cream. Mix mayonnaise and sour cream together. Add to pea mixture and toss. Chill well.

Joan Hyde
Yarmouth, Maine

Janet Richardson's
Party for Nana
May 7, 2011
Excellent
George says to add
pecans — great
summer salad

Watercress, Sweet Potato and Roasted Pecan Salad

"I love to eat lots of deep green vegetables. The sweet potato adds a perfect color accent! To make a complete lunch out of this salad, add thin-sliced strips of roasted free-range chicken."

Preparation Time: 20 minutes

4 servings

1 bunch watercress
1 medium sweet potato or yam, baked, then chilled
½ cup roasted pecan halves (5 to 10 minutes in 300° oven)

Lemon Vinaigrette
¼ cup extra virgin olive oil
¼ cup lemon juice or mild rice wine vinegar
1 teaspoon light honey
½ teaspoon tamari sauce
1 teaspoon Dijon mustard
¼ teaspoon minced garlic
¼ teaspoon each of some fresh herbs (thyme, oregano, basil, or
   your favorites)

Make vinaigrette first. Combine all vinaigrette ingredients and mix well. Set aside. Before untying watercress, trim bottom ½-inch off stems. Untie and remove yellowed or bruised leaves. Rinse well under cold running water, then cut stems in 1-inch sections, leaving upper leaves intact. Arrange watercress on each of 4 serving plates. Cut tips off sweet potato and peel off skin. Cut in half lengthwise; cut each half across in ¼-inch slices. Arrange slices on watercress. Stir vinaigrette and pour over salads. Top with pecan halves.

Vera Berv
Scarborough, Maine

Dorothy's Potato Salad

"My mother was always asked to bring this potato salad to potluck and church suppers in her hometown of Waterford, Maine. It is the best potato salad I have ever eaten. It is possible to substitute mayonnaise for the salad dressing, but never leave out the pickle juice! (Juice from homemade bread and butter pickles is best, but you can successfully use the "store bought" variety, if necessary.) The creamy texture and sweet-sour flavor can't be beat!"

Preparation Time: 30 minutes

8 to 10 servings

7	cups warm, boiled potatoes, peeled and cut in ½-inch dice
1	tablespoon very finely diced onion
1	teaspoon salt, or to taste
⅛	teaspoon pepper
1	tablespoon olive oil
½	cup plus 2 tablespoons juice from a jar of bread and butter pickles, divided
½	cup diced celery
½	cup diced cucumber
1½	cups Miracle Whip salad dressing
3	hard-boiled eggs
	Lettuce
	Cherry tomatoes
	Paprika

Combine warm potatoes, onion, salt, pepper, olive oil and 6 tablespoons of pickle juice. Mix gently, but well. Cover and chill for several hours or overnight. Just before serving mix together celery, cucumber, Miracle Whip, ¼ cup pickle juice and 2 chopped hard-boiled eggs. Combine dressing mixture and potato mixture. Mix well. Serve on bed of lettuce surrounded by cherry tomatoes. Garnish with slices of the remaining hard-boiled egg and sprinkle with paprika.

Kathleen Leslie
Cape Elizabeth, Maine

Vera's Brown Rice Salad

"I first ate this at "Patty and Ian's" wedding on Bustins Island. Ever since, it has been "my" salad and anyone who tastes it asks for the recipe."

Preparation Time: 30 minutes

10 servings

1   cup brown rice (I use Basmati), cooked in 1¾ cups water
      and cooled
1   cup cashews
¼   cup sesame seeds
¼   cup sunflower seeds
2   scallions, sliced
1   green bell pepper, diced
1   red bell pepper, diced
1   stalk celery, sliced
1   carrot, sliced
2   tablespoons minced parsley
½   cup raisins (optional)
1   cup bean sprouts (optional)
      Broccoli florets or watercress as garnish

Blender Dressing
¼   cup orange juice
½   cup vegetable oil (or ¼ cup vegetable oil and ¼ cup olive oil)
¼   cup tamari or soy sauce
1   tablespoon sesame oil
2   tablespoons dry sherry
      Juice of 1 lime
1   clove garlic
1   teaspoon fresh ginger

Toast nuts and seeds in hot (350°) oven for 8 minutes or until brown. Put all dressing ingredients in blender and whir until well mixed. Mix salad ingredients together. Pour dressing over salad. Toss and refrigerate at least 2 hours. Can make day ahead. Serve surrounded by broccoli florets or watercress.

Vera Berv
Scarborough, Maine

Rice Salad with Cilantro and Pine Nuts

"This is my version of a salad I tasted at the Museum of Fine Arts in Boston. I make this according to taste and looks, not on specific amounts of ingredients. Therefore all these measurements are adjustable."

Preparation Time: 30 minutes

8 servings

4	cups cooked rice
2	scallions, chopped
1	cup chopped cilantro
2	cups baby shrimp, cooked
½	3¼-ounce package gourmet sprouts
1	cup pine nuts
1	tablespoon olive oil
6	tablespoons rice wine vinegar
	Salt and pepper to taste

Toss together rice, scallions, cilantro, shrimp and sprouts. Brown pine nuts in olive oil, stirring often; add to salad. Toss salad with rice wine vinegar, salt and pepper.

Alice Spencer
Portland, Maine

Lentil Bulgur Salad

"This is a never fail dish for at home or potluck parties. People rave about this dish, which can be served as a meal, when accompanied by bread. Urge guests to squeeze lemon on it, especially if it's been in the fridge for a few days."

Preparation Time: 1 hour

6 servings

1	cup dry lentils
2	cups water
1	cup dry bulgur wheat, cracked
1	cup boiling water
¼	cup olive oil
¼	cup lemon juice
2	medium garlic cloves, crushed
1	teaspoon salt
½	teaspoon oregano
2	tablespoons minced fresh mint (or 2 teaspoons dried mint)
2-3	tablespoons minced fresh dill (or 2 to 3 teaspoons dried dill)
	Freshly ground black pepper, to taste
¼	cup minced fresh parsley, packed
⅓	cup finely minced onion
1	small bell pepper, any color, diced
½	stalk celery, finely minced
½	cup crumbled feta cheese
½	cup niçoise olives, a scant ¼ pound
1	medium tomato, diced
½	cup chopped, toasted walnuts
	Wedges of lemon

Place lentils in a medium saucepan, cover with 2 cups water and bring to boiling point. Turn heat way down, partially cover and allow to simmer, without agitation, for 20 to 25 minutes, or until lentils are tender but not mushy. Drain well and transfer to large bowl. While lentils cook, place the bulgur in a small bowl.
Add boiling water, cover and let stand 10 to 15 minutes. Add everything to lentils, except tomato, walnuts and lemon wedges.

Mix gently, but thoroughly. Cover tightly and refrigerate. Just before serving, top with tomatoes and walnuts. Garnish with lemon wedges.

Mary Lee Fowler
Pownal, Maine

Tortellini Salad

"This was a big hit with my daughter's boyfriend the first time he came to visit. It has become a favorite of theirs."

Preparation Time: 20 minutes

6 main dish servings

2	9-ounce packages refrigerated tortellini filled with cheese, mushroom or tomato
¼	cup basil flavored salad oil
¼	cup (or more) chopped onion
2	tablespoons balsamic vinegar
2	tablespoons chopped, fresh basil
1	tablespoon chopped, fresh oregano
1	tablespoon chopped, fresh chives
2	garlic cloves, minced
¼	teaspoon salt
⅛	teaspoon pepper
12-15	red cherry tomatoes
¾	cup pitted Kalamata black olives
¾	cup finely shredded Parmesan cheese
	Leaf lettuce
	Basil leaves for garnish

Cook tortellini according to package directions. Drain in colander and rinse in cold water, drain. In large bowl stir together oil, onion, vinegar, basil, oregano, chives, garlic, salt and pepper. Add tortellini, tomatoes, olives and cheese. Toss lightly to coat. Spoon onto lettuce; add basil garnish and serve. Can be made ahead and refrigerated. Bring to room temperature, adding cheese at the last moment.

Kay White
Portland, Maine

Pasta Pesto Florentine

Preparation Time: 15 minutes

8 servings

½   cup walnuts
2-3 cloves garlic
1   10-ounce package frozen chopped spinach, thawed
     and drained
½   cup Parmesan cheese
½   cup olive oil
⅓   cup water
1   teaspoon salt
1   teaspoon dried basil leaves
1   14-ounce pasta ruffles (tri-color is best), cooked and drained

Combine walnuts and garlic in blender until well chopped. Add spinach, Parmesan, oil, water, salt and basil. Blend until smooth. For thinner sauce stir in additional water. Spoon sauce over pasta; toss to coat well. Serve hot or cold.

Elizabeth Barnaby
Searsmont, Maine

Tester's Note: Quick and good. Would be nice to add fresh basil when available.

Pasta Peanut Salad

"Great with barbecued oriental style chicken."

Preparation Time: 20 minutes

4 servings

Salad
2   heaping cups dried bow-tie pasta
     Half a head of Chinese cabbage, coarsely chopped
       (4 to 6 cups)
1   medium red bell pepper cut into ¼-inch dice
4   large scallions, thinly sliced crosswise, using white and
       green parts
¾   cup unsalted, dry-roasted peanuts

Salad Dressing
½   cup natural peanut butter
¼   cup rice wine vinegar
3   tablespoons soy sauce
2   tablespoons honey
1   tablespoon Oriental sesame oil
¼   cup water
¾   teaspoon chili oil (more or less, according to taste)

Make salad dressing first. Whisk together peanut butter, vinegar, soy sauce, honey and sesame oil. Carefully blend in water. Keep stirring until smooth and creamy. Add chili oil according to taste. (Be careful, it's hot). Put aside ¼ cup of this dressing. Cook pasta until tender but still firm to the bite, about 12 minutes. Drain, then rinse with cold water and drain again. Transfer to large mixing bowl. Add vegetables and peanuts and mix carefully. Pour in the dressing and stir carefully until well mixed. Transfer to large serving bowl and serve with reserved dressing on side.

Margaret Wilkis
South Portland, Maine

Lemon-Garlic Penne with Asparagus and Pine Nuts

"This is everyone at Stonewall Kitchen Portland's favorite. Substitute broccoli or fresh snap peas for the asparagus. Great for picnics because it can stay out for hours without refrigeration."

Preparation Time: 25 minutes

6 to 8 servings

1   pound young asparagus, trimmed
8   ounces penne or rigatoni pasta
2-3 tablespoons fresh lemon juice
     Grated zest of one lemon
4-5 tablespoons Stonewall Kitchen Roasted Garlic Oil
4   tablespoons freshly grated Parmesan cheese
½   cup pine nuts, lightly toasted
     Salt and freshly ground black pepper to taste

Bring large pot of salted water to boil. Add asparagus and cook until tender, about 4 minutes. Remove asparagus with tongs; plunge into cold water to stop cooking. Blot dry and cut into 2-inch lengths. Boil pasta in same water until al dente. Drain; rinse under cold water and blot dry. Combine pasta and asparagus in a large bowl. Pour on lemon juice, zest and garlic oil and toss. Add Parmesan cheese, pine nuts, salt and plenty of black pepper. Toss again and serve.

Stonewall Kitchen
Portland, Maine

Pasta and Seafood Salad with Basil

Preparation Time: 30 minutes

6 to 8 servings

1	pound shrimp
1	pound bay scallops
½	pound pasta
1	cup tiny peas, uncooked
½	cup diced red pepper
½	cup minced Bermuda onion
½	cup olive oil
3-4	teaspoons lemon juice
½	cup basil pesto
	Salt and pepper to taste
1	cup black olives

Cook shrimp, scallops and pasta. Drain well and toss together. Add peas, pepper, onion and toss. Whisk together olive oil, lemon, basil, salt and pepper. Pour over seafood and pasta and toss well. Add black olives.

Judy Carter
Cape Elizabeth, Maine

Graduation Party Shrimp

Preparation Time: 45 minutes

6 servings

1	pound orzo, cooked
1	pound large shrimp, cooked and peeled
4	tablespoons olive oil, divided
4	ounces feta cheese, crumbled
1	large tomato, chopped
12	Kalamata olives, pitted
2	scallions, chopped
¼	cup fresh dill, minced
1½	cloves garlic, minced
3	tablespoons lemon juice
1½	tablespoons red wine vinegar
	Salt and pepper to taste

Toss orzo and shrimp with 1 tablespoon olive oil and chill 1 hour. Add rest of ingredients and chill 3 to 4 hours.

Connie Batson
Falmouth, Maine

Tofu Salad

"Very tasty and very healthy"

Preparation Time: 15 minutes

6 servings

½ pound tofu, drained and cubed
1 cup diced, cooked chicken
½ cup chopped celery
½ cup chopped scallions
½ cup chopped parsley
1½ cups halved green seedless grapes

Dressing
½ cup light mayonnaise
2 tablespoons lemon juice
2 tablespoons sour cream
2 tablespoons fresh tarragon
1 teaspoon Dijon mustard
½ teaspoon thyme

Combine salad ingredients. Mix dressing ingredients together.
Pour dressing over salad and toss thoroughly.

Maryanne Vitalius
Yarmouth, Maine

chicken Salad

"Our family has loved this recipe for 23 years. A dear friend first made it for me at a baby shower for our second daughter. Good food, good friends, good memories."

Preparation Time: 20 minutes

6 servings

1	quart cooked boneless chicken pieces
¼	cup sliced water chestnuts
½	pound seedless green grapes
½	cup chopped celery
½	cup toasted, slivered almonds
1	8-ounce can pineapple chunks, drained
¾	cup mayonnaise
1	teaspoon curry powder.
2	teaspoons soy sauce
2	teaspoons lemon juice
	Lettuce

Combine chicken, water chestnuts, grapes, celery, almonds and pineapple. Mix mayonnaise, curry, soy sauce and lemon juice in a bowl. Pour over chicken mixture. Toss lightly to mix and chill several hours. To serve, spoon on nests of lettuce.

Ann Kirner
Cape Elizabeth, Maine

Taco Salad

"A great summer salad for something different. Remember to prepare the salad in layers."

Preparation Time: 30 to 45 minutes

6 to 8 servings

2   pounds ground chuck
2   large packages taco seasoning
1½ cups water
1   bag restaurant-style taco chips
1   large head lettuce, chopped
2   large red onions, sliced thin
1   large can black olives, sliced
6   salad tomatoes, chopped
2   green peppers, chopped
1   12-ounce package shredded cheddar or Monterey Jack
     cheese
    Sour cream
    Avocado, chopped
    Salsa

Cook ground beef, drain, add taco seasoning and 1½ cups water. Simmer 10 to 15 minutes. Cool. In large bowl crush a handful of chips in bottom of bowl. Layer, over the chips, by the handful, meat, lettuce, onion, olives, tomatoes, peppers and cheese. Continue to layer ingredients, starting with chips, until all the ingredients are gone. Top salad with sour cream, avocado and salsa.

Marie Curtis
Farmington, New Hampshire

Watergate Salad

"This salad takes '18 minutes' to make and the cool whip 'covers everything up', hence the name 'Watergate Salad'."

Preparation Time: 18 minutes

6 servings

1   3⅛-ounce package instant pistachio pudding
1   20-ounce can crushed pineapple (do not drain)
1   8- or 9-ounce container frozen whipped topping
⅓   10½-ounce package mini marshmallows

Mix all ingredients and chill until firm.

Harriet Currie
Yarmouth, Maine

Dot's Molded Salad

Preparation Time: 15 minutes

6 servings

1   3-ounce package raspberry gelatin
1   16-ounce can whole cranberry sauce
1   8-ounce can crushed pineapple

Mix gelatin in 1 cup of hot water and stir 2 minutes. Stir in cranberries and pineapple, juice and all. Mix until well blended. Chill in refrigerator overnight. Serve with whipped topping if desired.

Louise T. Berry
Island Falls, Maine

Tester's Note: Tastes and looks like a childhood memory.

Entrées

Meat, Poultry & Seafood

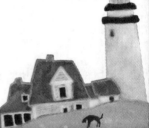

Beef Tips with a Twist

Preparation Time: 15 minutes

Cooking Time: 20 minutes

6 servings

1   tablespoon olive oil (garlic flavored)
3   small top round steaks or moose meat steak (shoulder)
1   medium onion, sliced
1   cup cut-up broccoli
1   cup sliced shiitake mushrooms, stems removed
1   cup brewed tea, green or black
    Parsley, to taste
    Thyme, to taste
    Dried basil, to taste

Slice steak into cubes. In a skillet, sauté beef and onions in olive oil until beef is brown on both sides. Add vegetables and tea. Simmer 10 minutes. Add seasonings and simmer until juices have reduced. It may be necessary to add ½ cup water or more as shiitake mushrooms absorb water. Serve with rice.

Audrey Joy
Belfast, Maine

Beef Burgundy

Preparation Time: 45 to 60 minutes

Cooking Time: 1½ hours

10 to 12 servings

1	pound peeled small white onions
6	strips bacon, diced
¼	cup margarine or butter
4	pounds beef cubes
¼	cup brandy (optional)
1½	teaspoons salt
¼	teaspoon fresh ground pepper
2	cups burgundy or other dry red wine
2	peeled garlic cloves
2	cups small whole or sliced mushrooms
1½	cups water
1-2	sprigs parsley
1	celery top
1	carrot, quartered
1	bay leaf
1	teaspoon dried thyme or 1 tablespoon fresh thyme
6	tablespoons flour
½	cup cold water

Brown onions and bacon in margarine in Dutch oven. Remove and set aside. Brown meat in same Dutch oven. If desired, pour brandy over and set aflame. Add salt and pepper to meat. Add burgundy, garlic, mushrooms, 1½ cups water, onions and bacon to meat. Make a bouquet garni by tying together parsley, celery top, carrot, bay leaf and thyme in a piece of cheesecloth. Use long string for easy removal later. Add to mixture. Cover and simmer 1½ hours. Remove beef, mushrooms and onions and arrange in casserole. Strain liquid, discarding garlic, bacon and bouquet garni. Mix flour and ½ cup water to a smooth paste. Add to meat stock, stirring until gravy is thick and smooth. Add to meat and mushroom mixture. Serve immediately or refrigerate. To reheat: bake in covered casserole dish at 350° for 35 minutes.

Andy Beauchesne
Peru, Maine

Green Pepper Steak

"The origin of this recipe is unknown; however, it is quick and tasty and I make it often."

Preparation Time: 20 minutes

Cooking Time: 40 minutes

4 servings

1	pound round or flank steak, fat trimmed
¼	cup soy sauce
1	clove garlic
½	teaspoon ground ginger or 1½ teaspoons fresh grated ginger
¼	cup oil
1	cup thinly sliced green onion,
1	cup red and/or green peppers, cut in 1-inch squares
2	stalks thinly sliced celery
1	tablespoon cornstarch
1	cup water
2	tomatoes, cut in wedges

Cut beef across grain into thin strips, ⅛-inch thick. Combine soy sauce, garlic and ginger. Add beef. Toss and set aside. Heat oil in fry pan or wok. Add beef and toss over high heat until brown. Cover and simmer on low heat for 30 minutes or until tender. Turn up heat and add sliced vegetables. Toss until tender and crisp, about 10 minutes. Mix cornstarch with water and add to pan. Cook, stirring, until thickened. Add tomatoes and heat through.

Dee Dole
Portland, Maine

Tester's Note: Good served with rice.

Stuffed Burgers

Preparation Time: 20 minutes

Grilling Time: 12 minutes

4 servings

1½ pounds ground beef
1¼ teaspoons salt
¼ teaspoon pepper
⅔ cup shredded zucchini
⅓ cup thinly sliced mushrooms
¼ cup chopped red pepper
½ teaspoon Italian seasonings
2 tablespoons olive oil
2 tablespoons grated Parmesan cheese
4 whole wheat hamburger buns
4 teaspoons butter (optional)

Sprinkle 1 teaspoon salt and pepper over ground beef; mix lightly but thoroughly. Divide meat into 8 equal portions and form into thin patties. In olive oil, cook zucchini, mushrooms, red pepper, Italian seasonings and remaining salt in large frying pan over medium heat 3 to 4 minutes, stirring occasionally. Cool. Stir in Parmesan cheese. Place equal amounts of vegetable mixture in center of meat patties. Top with remaining patties. Press edges together securely to seal. Grill over medium coals 5 to 6 minutes. Turn and grill for 5 to 6 minutes. If desired, spread butter on each bun and grill for 1 minute.

Market Square Health Care Center
South Paris, Maine

Tester's Note: A variety of vegetables could be added to the hamburg making this a versatile dish.

Meatloaf

"This was one of the few recipes I have that belonged to my mother. She was not a cook. Her idea of baking a pie was to buy a frozen one and put it in the oven. However, her meatloaf is the best I have ever had; it's very moist and the tomato sauce adds just the right flavor."

Preparation Time: 15 minutes

Baking Time: 1 to 1½ hours

6 to 8 servings

3	pounds ground meat, preferably ⅓ each of beef, pork and veal (can use all beef)
¾	cup chopped celery
¾	cup chopped onion
2	slices white bread, torn apart
¾	cup milk
1-2	eggs, beaten
1½	teaspoons baking powder
	Salt to taste
	Pepper to taste
	Celery salt to taste
1	8-ounce can tomato sauce

Preheat oven to 350°. Mix ground meats together. Using your hands, mix all other ingredients with meat, except tomato sauce. Form into loaf and place in 9x13-inch pan. Bake for 1 to 1½ hours. During last 20 minutes, pour tomato sauce over meatloaf.

Polly Pierce
Portland, Maine

Newton's Meatloaf

"This was Newton's favorite which he prepared for the family or church pot luck suppers."

Preparation Time: 15 minutes

Baking Time: 1 to 1½ hours

1 large loaf

1½ pounds ground beef
1   onion, chopped
½   8-ounce can tomato sauce
1½ teaspoons salt
1   cup bread crumbs
1   egg, beaten
½   teaspoon pepper

Sauce
½   8-ounce can tomato sauce
1   cup water
2   tablespoons prepared mustard
2   tablespoons vinegar
2   tablespoons brown sugar

Preheat oven to 350°. Mix all the meatloaf ingredients together. Place meatloaf in 9½x5½-inch loaf pan. Combine sauce ingredients and pour over meatloaf. Bake for 1 to 1½ hours, basting occasionally.

Joyce A. Lamb for Newton S. Lamb
West Paris, Maine

Sassy Meatloaf

Preparation Time: 15 minutes

Baking Time: 1 hour and 5 minutes

6 servings

1	pound lean ground beef
1¼	cups salsa
¾	cup quick oatmeal
1	carrot, shredded
2	plum tomatoes, diced
½	cup coarsely chopped mushrooms

Preheat oven to 325°. Mix all of the above together. Spray a 9x4-inch or 9x5-inch loaf pan lightly with nonstick spray. Fill pan with above mixture. Cook about 1 hour and 5 minutes or until meatloaf begins to brown.

Krista Martin
Westbrook, Maine

Meatballs and Mushroom Gravy

"As my husband's dementia became more acute, his appetite diminished and it took him a very long time to eat. I found that recipes that were easy to eat were more appealing to him and had a better chance of getting eaten. Because they were quick was an added appeal to me."

Preparation Time: 20 minutes

Cooking Time: 30 minutes

4 servings

1	pound ground beef
½	teaspoon salt
⅛	teaspoon pepper
⅛	teaspoon celery salt
⅛	teaspoon garlic powder
½	cup bread crumbs
½	cup water
2	tablespoons onion, diced small

Gravy

1	can mushroom soup
¼	can water
1	tablespoon gravy coloring

Combine meatball ingredients together and mix well. Shape into meatballs. Broil to brown or sauté in pan until brown on all sides. Mix soup, water and gravy coloring until smooth and add meatballs. Simmer for 30 minutes. Serve over rice.

Marjorie Jamback
Biddeford, Maine

Tester's Note: Sliced mushrooms, or wine can be added to the gravy. Also, a little sage or thyme added to the meat mixture gives a little different flavoring.

Swedish Meatballs

"This recipe was given to me about 50 years ago by a good neighbor. It has become a family favorite."

Preparation Time: 30 minutes

Cooking Time: 1 hour

20 meatballs

2	slices bread
½	cup milk (scant)
1	pound ground beef
1	egg, beaten
	Salt and pepper to taste
	Flour, for rolling meatballs
	Oil, for browning meatballs
1	16-ounce can tomatoes
	Water, enough to cover meatballs
1	large onion, sliced

Moisten bread in milk and beat with fork. Add beef, egg, salt and pepper and mix well. Make small balls and roll in flour. Brown in a little oil in fry pan. Transfer to large saucepan and cover with can of tomatoes. Add water to cover and put in onion. Simmer 1 hour or longer.

Lois S. Grant
Kennebunkport, Maine

Tester's Note: ¼ teaspoon nutmeg and/or a little browned onion added to the meatballs could be included for additional flavor.

Italian Zucchini and Beef

"My papa (grandfather) owns an Italian restaurant. This recipe has been handed down for 3 generations. Living in a Polish-Italian home, we always had great meals, said my mother. My mother and grandmother both died of Alzheimer's, but all their handwritten recipes live on."

Preparation Time: 20 to 30 minutes

Baking Time: 40 to 50 minutes

6 to 8 servings

4   medium zucchini, sliced ¼-inch lengthwise
     Salt and pepper to taste

Sauce
1   pound ground beef
1   small onion, chopped
4   medium tomatoes, peeled and sliced
2   cups tomato sauce
½   teaspoon oregano
½   teaspoon basil
¼   teaspoon rosemary

Cheese Filling
1   cup ricotta cheese
1   cup small curd cottage cheese
2   eggs
4   ounces Provolone cheese, sliced or grated
4   ounces mozzarella cheese, sliced or grated
⅓   cup Parmesan cheese

Preheat oven to 375°. Steam zucchini. In large skillet, sauté beef and onion. Drain off fat. Add tomatoes, tomato sauce and seasonings. Simmer uncovered for 15 minutes, stirring occasionally. Grease 9x13-inch pan or dish. Arrange half of slices of zucchini on bottom and sprinkle with salt and pepper. If zucchini are too long, cut in half. Blend ricotta, cottage cheese and eggs. Spread ½ mixture over zucchini. Add ½ of Provolone and mozzarella and ½ of sauce. Repeat these layers. Top with Parmesan cheese. Bake 40 to 50 minutes.

Catherine A. Churchill
Bar Harbor, Maine

zucchini Stroganoff

"This is a one-pan meal and a great way to use zucchini."

Preparation Time: 30 minutes

Cooking Time: 30 to 45 minutes

2 servings

½	pound ground beef
¼	cup onion, chopped
½	can mushroom soup
1	cup uncooked egg noodles
1	zucchini, sliced
	Salt and pepper to taste
½	teaspoon chervil or basil
⅔	cup sour cream

Cook ground beef and onion in skillet. Cook until beef loses its pink color. Add rest of ingredients except sour cream. Simmer covered until noodles are done. Add sour cream and warm through. Other ground meats may be used with various spices. Try pork sausage with savory or marjoram, lamb with basil or oregano, or veal with rosemary or tarragon.

Valerie Howard
Hulls Cove, Maine

Meat-Cabbage Casserole

"We used to prepare Finnish stuffed cabbage rolls growing up, but this is much easier to make and tastes very much like the old version."

Preparation Time: 30 minutes

Baking Time: 1 hour

6 to 8 servings

1	medium cabbage, shredded
2	tablespoons butter
2	tablespoons dark corn syrup
2	teaspoons salt
¼	teaspoon ground marjoram
1	pound lean ground beef
1	cup bread crumbs
½	cup milk
2	eggs, beaten

Preheat oven to 350°. Cook cabbage in enough boiling water to cover for about 5 minutes or just until tender. Drain. Place in bowl. Add butter, syrup, salt and marjoram to cabbage. In another bowl, mix ground beef, bread crumbs, milk and eggs. Butter a 2-quart casserole and layer cabbage and meat mixture, beginning and ending with cabbage. Bake for 1 hour, or until meat is done.

Carol Jamback Weldin
Andover, Massachusetts

stuffed cabbage

"This recipe is given in memory of my mother, Marie Ange Michaud Dunn."

Preparation Time: 45 minutes

Baking Time: 2½ hours

16 medium rolls

1	large head cabbage
3	pounds ground beef
⅔	cup rice, uncooked
1	large onion, chopped
1	12-ounce can tomato sauce
1	teaspoon salt
1	teaspoon pepper

Sauce

1	30-ounce can tomatoes
2	18-ounce cans tomato sauce

Preheat oven to 350°. Steam cabbage leaves. Mix hamburg, rice, onion, tomato sauce, salt and pepper. Place heaping spoonful meat mixture in each cabbage leaf and wrap like package; secure with toothpick. Place rolls in roasting pan and top with canned tomatoes and tomato sauce. Bake for 2½ hours or until tender.

Marion Bourgoin
Frenchville, Maine

Picadillo

"There are different ways to make this traditional Mexican dish. I make it often, using lots of hot sauce."

Preparation Time: 30 minutes

Cooking Time: 30 minutes

4 servings

1	medium onion, minced
1	clove garlic, minced
4	tablespoons oil
2	fresh tomatoes, peeled and chopped
2	cups chopped cooked beef or ground beef
½	cup beef stock
¼	cup raisins (optional)
1	teaspoon vinegar
1	pinch cloves
1	small pinch cumin
	Salt and pepper to taste
	Hot sauce (optional)

Fry onion and garlic in oil for about 5 minutes. Add chopped tomatoes and meat, stirring ingredients well. Add beef stock and remaining ingredients. Simmer about 30 minutes. This makes very good stuffing for tamales or tacos. You can also make a burrito with flour tortilla.

Anna Lujan
Montebello, California

Liver and Mushrooms with Wine Sauce

"The only way I like liver. Sometimes I use more than the 5 mushrooms. Can be served with rice or mashed potatoes."

Preparation Time: 20 minutes

Cooking Time: 15 minutes

4 servings

2	tablespoons butter
2	tablespoons oil
1	small onion, chopped fine
5	mushrooms, chopped
	Flour
	Salt
	Pepper
2	pounds beef liver, cut into small pieces
¼	cup red wine

Melt butter in fry pan with oil. Add onion and mushrooms and sauté. Mix flour with salt and pepper. Coat liver pieces in seasoned flour. Push vegetables to side of pan and add liver. Cook 4 minutes on each side. Remove meat to serving dish. Add wine to vegetables and mix with pan juices. Pour over meat on serving dish.

Charlotte LaCrosse
Rockland, Maine

Teriyaki Marinade for Flank Steak

Preparation Time: 15 minutes

Marinating Time: 4 hours or overnight

1 cup

⅓	cup soy sauce
⅓	cup brown sugar
⅓	cup oil
1	tablespoon onion, chopped fine
½	tablespoon ginger, freshly grated
2	garlic cloves
2	bay leaves
½	cup pineapple juice

Process all ingredients for 10 seconds. Put meat in marinade; turn regularly before grilling. Marinate a minimum of 4 hours. Overnight is preferred.

Churchill Caterers & Event Planners
Portland, Maine

Sou Tse Tofu

Preparation Time: 20 minutes

Cooking Time: 10 minutes

2 to 3 servings

2	tablespoons oil
2	tablespoons minced green onion
½	tablespoon minced garlic clove
½	teaspoon minced ginger root
¼	pound ground beef, pork or chicken
¼	teaspoon sugar
1	tablespoon cooking wine
2½	tablespoons soy sauce
2	teaspoons cornstarch
¾	cup stock or water
½	pound tofu, cut into small pieces
2	tablespoons chopped fresh garlic or green onion
	Dash of Szechwan peppercorn powder (optional)

Heat oil. Stir fry onion, garlic and ginger root in oil until fragrant. Add ground meat; stir until meat is cooked and separated. Combine sugar, cooking wine, soy sauce, cornstarch, stock or water and tofu in bowl and add to meat mixture. Bring to boil, stirring until sauce thickens (about 3 minutes). Sprinkle with fresh garlic or green onion and Szechwan peppercorn. Serve.

John Leslie
Sante Fe, New Mexico

Tester's Note: Also good served with shrimp.

The Best Barbecued Baby Back Ribs

"Although this recipe takes a while to make, it is worth it. This is a special family treat."

Preparation Time: 30 minutes

Cooking Time: 2 hours 30 minutes

6 servings

4	cups beer
2	cups root beer
2½	cups dark brown sugar
1½	cups apple cider vinegar
1½	tablespoons chili powder
1½	tablespoons ground cumin
1	tablespoon dry mustard
2	teaspoons salt
2	teaspoons dried crushed red pepper
2	bay leaves
6	pounds baby back pork ribs, cut into 4 rib sections

Preheat oven to 325°. Line jelly roll pan with foil. Bring first 10 ingredients to a boil in very large pot. Reduce heat. Simmer 1 minute to blend flavors. Add half of ribs to sauce. Cover pot and simmer until ribs are tender, turning frequently, about 25 minutes. (Sauce should be boiling lightly). Place ribs on foil-lined pan and cover lightly with foil. Then, repeat simmering with rest of ribs and add to other ribs on jelly roll pan. Crimp foil over sides of pan and bake for ½ hour. Boil barbecue sauce, uncovered on medium to medium high heat until reduced to about 3 cups. This should take about 40 minutes to 1 hour. It will thicken significantly. This will be the barbecue sauce with which to baste the ribs. Brush ribs with sauce and salt according to taste. Put on preheated grill (medium heat) until heated through and glazed. The ribs should be cooked throughout by the time they are barbecued so don't over-grill, about 15 minutes, depending on personal preference. Serve with extra warm sauce on the side.

Margaret Wilkis
Cape Elizabeth, Maine

Pork Chops

Preparation Time: 10 minutes

Baking Time: 1½ hours

4 to 6 servings

4-6 medium thick pork chops
½   teaspoon nutmeg
½   teaspoon celery seed
1   bay leaf, crumbled
½   cup catsup
¼   cup vinegar
1   cup water

Preheat oven to 325°. Brown chops in skillet on both sides. Place in casserole dish. Mix remaining ingredients together and pour over chops. Cover and bake for 1½ hours.

Joan Hyde
Yarmouth, Maine

Pork à la Frim Fram

Preparation Time: 30 minutes

Cooking Time: 5 to 10 minutes

2 servings

1	tablespoon butter
⅓	cup chopped ginger root
⅓	cup minced garlic
⅓	cup chopped peanuts
¼	teaspoon red curry paste
¼	cup cream of coconut
¼	cup pineapple juice
	Cornstarch (optional)
1	teaspoon soy sauce
1	pork tenderloin (roasted, grilled or cooked as you wish), sliced

In small sauce pan, heat butter. Stir in ginger, garlic, peanuts and curry paste. Add cream of coconut, pineapple juice and soy sauce. You may thicken with cornstarch, if desired. Put sauce on each plate. Arrange slices of pork on top and serve.

Michael Myers, Innkeeper
Lake House
Waterford, Maine

Polish Pig in Blanket

"This recipe was passed on to my sister by her Hungarian friend in Florida. Mrs. Chomey is adamant about only using ground pork for this recipe. My sister had 3 children, all with different tastes. But they all loved this recipe which is big enough for a family get-together."

Preparation Time: 30 to 45 minutes

Baking Time: 2 hours

10 to 12 servings

Cabbage Rolls
1½ cups cooked rice
1 head cabbage
2 pounds fresh ground pork
1½ pounds ground ham
2 medium to large onions, chopped
3 cloves garlic, minced
2 tablespoons shortening or butter
4 eggs, beaten
 Salt and pepper to taste
2 cans sauerkraut

Gravy
2 tablespoons shortening or butter
2 tablespoons flour
2 cups hot water
1 teaspoon caraway seeds (optional)
 Sugar and salt to taste
½ cup tomato juice

Preheat oven to 350°. Boil cabbage until leaves are softened. Mix meats, chopped onion and sauté with garlic in 2 tablespoons shortening or butter. Add beaten eggs, salt, pepper and rice. Place a little of mixture in each cabbage leaf and roll up. Place ½ of sauerkraut on bottom of big pan (Dutch Oven). Place cabbage rolls on this layer of sauerkraut. Top with remaining sauerkraut. To make gravy; mix shortening or butter, flour, 2 cups hot water, caraway seeds, sugar, salt and tomato juice. Prick cabbage rolls with knife or fork and pour gravy over top. Bake for 2 hours.

Marjorie Fuller
South Paris, Maine

Jambalaya

"This recipe is from my 90 year old great aunt, who likes hot, spicy food. Recipe especially good on a cold day after skiing or snowmobiling."

Preparation Time: 1½ hours

Cooking Time: 35 to 50 minutes

8 servings

1	pound country sausage
1	large onion, chopped
1	teaspoon garlic powder
2	medium green peppers, chopped
3	hot peppers (habanero, chile or jalepeño), chopped
1	cup celery cut into ½-inch slices
1	pound fully-cooked ham, cut up in 1-inch cubes
1	15-ounce can tomatoes, cut up
1	pound frozen cleaned shrimp, thawed
1	11-ounce can tomato paste
1	teaspoon chili powder
1	teaspoon thyme
1	teaspoon basil

Using a large, deep skillet, sauté first 6 ingredients. Add all other ingredients. Heat until blended for 35 to 50 minutes. Serve over rice or noodles. Omit hot peppers for milder taste.

Kathy Warman
Portland, Maine

Bugullion

"This easy recipe with the odd name appeared in my brother's Boy Scout Handbook in the 1930's, and has been a family favorite ever since. It is excellent for a camp-out and has pleased groups of American Girl Scouts as well as Venezuelan Girl Guides. It has even been prepared high in the Andes on the tailgate of a station wagon over a sterno stove, while the cold mists swirled about us."

Preparation Time: 5 minutes

Cooking Time: 15 minutes

> Onions
> Hot dogs
> Baked beans
> Corn

Brown onions. Add sliced hot dogs, baked beans and corn and heat through.

Shirley Corse
Scarborough, Maine

Tester's Note: Use amounts of each item to suit your taste. Easy and tasty for a camping trip.

Garlic-Roasted Lamb

"A meal my mom would always make at Easter. It is a nice dinner for any special occasion. Sometimes I flavor the lamb by covering it with lemon slices before roasting."

Preparation Time: 20 minutes

Roasting Time: 1½ to 2 hours

6 servings

1	shank half leg lamb (about 3 pounds)
8	cloves garlic, sliced in half lengthwise
2	large sprigs fresh rosemary or 2 teaspoons dried
2	teaspoons olive oil
4	large sweet potatoes, peeled and cut into 1-inch cubes
6	parsnips, cut into 1-inch pieces
⅛	teaspoon salt
⅛	teaspoon pepper
1	lemon, cut into slices (optional)

Preheat oven to 325°. With sharp knife, trim the fat and cartilage from lamb. Season with salt and pepper. With small knife, make slits about 1-inch deep over lamb. Stuff each slit with garlic half and rosemary leaves. In large roasting pan, combine oil with sweet potatoes, parsnips and any remaining garlic. Coat well. Move vegetables to side of pan and place lamb in center. Season with salt and pepper. Place lemon slices on lamb. Roast in oven for about 1½ to 2 hours or until meat thermometer reads 160° (cooked medium). Turn the vegetables, occasionally, while roasting for even cooking. Remove pan from oven. With slotted spoon, place vegetables on serving dish and keep warm. Place lamb on carving platter; cover with foil and let stand 5 minutes. Slice the roast lamb and serve with vegetables.

SuSu DePaolo
South Portland, Maine

Braised Lamb and Eggplant

"This recipe was introduced to us by an Iranian exchange student. We felt "akin" to each other from our first bite and it has become a favorite dish of our family. Though our exchange student has been gone for over twenty years, it is still a favorite and we think of him when we eat this meal."

Preparation Time: 1 hour

Cooking Time: 2½ hours

4 servings

1	medium eggplant, 1 to 1½ pounds
¼	cup salt
1	quart water
¾	cup olive oil, divided
1	medium onion, peeled and cut into ¼-inch slices
1½	pounds lean boneless lamb shoulder, cut into 2-inch cubes
½	teaspoon turmeric
2	cups beef stock
2	tablespoons tomato paste
1	teaspoon salt
	Freshly ground pepper
1	medium tomato, cut crosswise into 4 slices
2	tablespoons fresh lemon juice
1	tablespoon bottled pomegranate syrup (optional)

Peel and slice eggplant lengthwise into 8 long strips. At room temperature, soak eggplant for 10 minutes in 1 quart water with ¼ cup salt. Meanwhile, heat ¼ cup olive oil on moderate heat, add onions and cook 10 minutes until brown. Set aside. Drain eggplant; pat dry. Heat ¼ cup oil and add eggplant, browning on all sides. Set aside. In remaining oil, brown lamb cubes seasoned with turmeric. Add stock, tomato paste, 1 teaspoon salt and ground pepper. Bring to boil, removing any scum that may cling to pan. Add browned onions and reduce heat to low. Simmer tightly covered for 45 minutes. Arrange eggplant side by side on top of lamb. Place tomato slices on top of eggplant. Pour in lemon juice and pomegranate syrup. Cover tightly and simmer

45 minutes more or until eggplant and lamb are tender. Season to taste and serve immediately. Serve with rice.

Barbara Payson
Falmouth, Maine

Tester's Note: If using canned beef stock, you may want to reduce amount of salt.

Leg of Lamb

Preparation Time: 30 minutes

Cooking Time: 4 hours

8 servings

1	5-pound leg of lamb
¼	cup oil
1	cup water
	Meat tenderizer
	Celery salt
1	onion, sliced
6	potatoes, cut into large pieces (or small whole new potatoes)
4	large carrots, cut into pieces

Remove skin from lamb. In heavy pan, brown lamb on all sides in oil. Add water to pan and cover, cooking for 1 hour over very low heat. Turn meat occasionally adding small amount of water as needed. Do not let pan cook dry. After 1 hour, pat lamb with meat tenderizer and celery salt. Place sliced onion on top of lamb and cook, covered, on low heat for 2 hours, adding more water if necessary. Add potatoes and carrots. Continue to cook for 1 more hour. Serve on platter.

Connie Gagne
Biddeford, Maine

Lamb Shanks à la Greque

Preparation Time: 15 minutes

Cooking Time: 3 hours

4 servings

4   lamb shanks (about 1 pound each)
2   tablespoons olive oil
2   cups beef bouillon
1-2 tablespoons lemon juice
½   teaspoon oregano
½   teaspoon thyme
½   teaspoon rosemary
1   bay leaf
     Salt and pepper, to taste

Brown shanks on all sides in olive oil over medium heat. Drain off fat, lower heat and add remaining ingredients. Cover and simmer 2 to 2½ hours until meat is tender when pierced with fork. Skim off any more fat that collects. Remove meat and keep warm while boiling down liquid to thicken gravy. Serve with cooked rice with lemon gravy on side.

John Gale, M.D.
Gloucester, Massachusetts

Mint Sauce for Lamb

"This subtle mint sauce works with lamb of any cut or preparation."

Preparation Time: 20 minutes

Cooking Time: 20 minutes

9 to 10 servings

¾ cup sliced shallots
2 tablespoons butter
2 cups beef broth
1 cup chopped mint
¾ cup red wine vinegar
½ cup sugar
1 tablespoon cornstarch

Sauté shallots in butter and add broth, reserving ¼ cup. Add chopped mint to broth/shallot mixture. Add vinegar and sugar and bring to boil. Add cornstarch that has been combined with ¼ cup of broth and simmer until desired thickness.

Michael Myers, Innkeeper
Lake House
Waterford, Maine

Tester's Note: This recipe can be halved and will yield 1⅛ cups to serve 4 to 5.

Aegean Chicken

Preparation Time: 30 to 40 minutes

Cooking Time: 30 minutes

6 servings

4-5 boneless, skinned chicken breasts cut into large pieces
1 9-ounce jar marinated artichoke hearts (drain and reserve liquid)
¼ cup olive oil, divided
    Flour to dredge chicken
½ pound quartered mushrooms
2-3 tablespoons butter
1 22-ounce can Italian tomatoes with liquid
3 cloves minced garlic
1 teaspoon salt
¾ teaspoon pepper
¾ teaspoon oregano
1 teaspoon basil
½ cup pitted olives
¾ cup cooking sherry

Preheat oven to 350°. Combine half artichoke liquid with 2 teaspoons olive oil in large, heavy-bottom frying pan. Dredge chicken in flour. Sauté in pan in batches, adding more artichoke liquid if needed. Remove and set aside. Sauté mushrooms in same pan, adding butter as needed. Remove and set aside. Pour tomatoes with liquid, garlic, and seasonings into pan and simmer 10 minutes. Add chicken, olives, mushrooms, artichokes and sherry. Cook 10 minutes. Pour into baking dish and heat until bubbly. Serve over rice or orzo.

Barbara Thelin
Cape Elizabeth, Maine

Note: This recipe can be refrigerated or frozen.

Amish Style Chicken Casserole

"This is a recipe I use most often when taking dinner to a family with a sick member, or a family just returning from a long trip. It is very easy to prepare and freezes well."

Preparation Time: 30 minutes

Baking Time: 20 minutes

6 to 8 servings

8	ounces egg noodles
½	cup butter or margarine
1	cup thinly sliced mushrooms
⅓	cup flour
2	cups chicken broth (canned will do)
1	cup milk
¼	cup pimiento, cut into strips
2	teaspoons salt
½	teaspoon pepper
2	cups cut-up cooked chicken
⅓	cup grated Parmesan cheese

Preheat oven to 350°. Cook noodles according to package directions and drain. In large skillet, melt butter and sauté mushrooms. Blend in flour. Gradually add broth, milk, pimiento, salt and pepper, stirring constantly until sauce is thickened. Add other ingredients, except noodles, and blend. In greased, 2½ quart casserole, combine noodles, chicken and sauce. Top with cheese. Bake 20 minutes.

Edith Farnum
Freeport, Maine

173

Blackened Chicken

Preparation Time: 10 minutes plus marinating time

Cooking Time: 10 minutes

4 servings

1	8-ounce bottle Italian dressing
½	cup dry white wine
4	skinless, boneless chicken breasts
1	tablespoon ground marjoram
1	tablespoon oregano
1	tablespoon thyme
1	teaspoon salt
1	teaspoon black pepper
½	teaspoon ground cayenne pepper
½	cup melted butter

Combine dressing and wine and marinate chicken for at least
1 hour. Combine all spices. Spread spice mixture on plate. Heat
12-inch skillet over high heat until smoking (5 to 10 minutes).
Drain chicken and dip into seasonings, coating both sides. Place in
hot skillet. Pour 2 tablespoons butter over each piece. Reduce heat
to medium. Cook 3 to 5 minutes on each side until cooked.

Colleen Gurney
Mexico, Maine

Broiled Maple Orange Chicken Breasts

"Yum! Easy and quick for an everyday meal, or your special guest. It is sure to become one of your favorites."

Preparation Time: 15 minutes (after marinating all night)

Broiling Time: 16 to 18 minutes

4 servings

⅓	cup Stonewall Kitchen Maine Maple Champagne Mustard
¼	cup fresh orange juice
	Grated zest of 1 large orange
2	tablespoons Stonewall Kitchen Roasted Garlic Oil
2	teaspoons Worcestershire sauce
1	tablespoon minced flat-leaf parsley
	Plus additional parsley for garnish
	Freshly ground black pepper to taste
2	medium whole chicken breasts, bone in, rinsed and patted dry

Stir together Maine Maple Champagne Mustard, orange juice and zest, Roasted Garlic Oil, Worcestershire sauce, parsley and pepper in a bowl. Pour into a large zip-top plastic bag; add chicken breasts, turning to cover well. Refrigerate for at least 4 hours or overnight, turning once or twice. Heat broiler. Place breasts flesh side down in shallow baking pan and spoon some of the marinade over them. Broil about 6 to 7 inches from heat for about 9 to 10 minutes. Turn, spoon over remaining marinade, and cook until breast meat is done and skin is browned, 7 to 8 minutes. Remove and allow to stand for 5 minutes. Dribble on remaining parsley and serve.

Stonewall Kitchen
Portland, Maine

Note: Skin can be removed and breast split, if desired.

Busy Day Chicken

"This is an old stand-by for many, but was my mother's staple recipe for church dinners, casseroles for friends in need, dinner for the family after a hectic day, or for unexpected guests. It has become the same for me. My mother bought inexpensive wine just for the casserole. I use any opened bottle. This is a very casual recipe. I have made the casserole and left it unbaked in the refrigerator all day before baking it."

Preparation Time: 20 minutes

Baking Time: 1 to 1½ hours

4 to 6 servings

6	skinned chicken pieces
1	10¾-ounce can cream of mushroom soup
1	cup uncooked white rice
21½	ounces (2 soup cans) white wine
21½	ounces (2 soup cans) water
1	package onion soup mix
	Sprinkle of paprika

Preheat oven to 350°. Place chicken in baking dish. Mix all remaining ingredients, except paprika, together and pour over chicken. Sprinkle with paprika. Bake for 1 to 1½ hours until all liquid is absorbed.

Gail Dransfield
Cape Elizabeth, Maine

chicken cacciatore

"This is my husband's favorite dish, first made for him by his mother, who now has Alzheimer's disease. She used a whole stick of butter, but I find that using half olive oil and half butter lends almost all the wonderful flavor. It is best made ahead, and the leftover sauce is great for another meal."

Preparation Time: 30 minutes

Cooking Time: 35 to 45 minutes

5 servings

4 tablespoons olive oil
4 tablespoons butter (½ stick)
2 diced large onions
2 diced green peppers
1 chicken (3½ to 4 pounds) cut into 8 pieces, or 4 boneless thighs and 4 boneless breast halves
3-4 thinly sliced cloves of garlic
1 16-ounce can stewed tomatoes (about 2 cups)
1 15-ounce can tomato sauce (1¾ to 2 cups)
2 bay leaves
1 teaspoon crushed, dried oregano
1 teaspoon salt
½ teaspoon celery seed
¼ teaspoon freshly ground pepper
4 scrubbed and quartered potatoes
½ cup dry red wine

In a large, deep skillet, sauté onions and peppers in oil and butter until soft, about 5 minutes. With slotted spoon, remove vegetables to bowl. Add chicken and brown on all sides. Toward the end of this process, add sliced garlic and brown. Return vegetables to pan and add stewed tomatoes, tomato sauce, bay leaves, oregano, salt, celery seed, pepper and potatoes and stir well. Cover, reduce heat to low and simmer until chicken is cooked through and sauce is thick, about 35 to 45 minutes. Slowly pour wine into the skillet and stir to combine. Cook for 2 minutes more and serve.

Patricia Noonan
Purchase, New York

Tester's Note: The leftovers, served over pasta make an easy meal.

Chicken Marsala

"This is our family favorite. It can be made to serve 2 or 80. The recipe is very reliable. We have used it for birthday gatherings, anniversaries and intimate dinners for two! Mushrooms and chicken can be prepared in advance. Just combine all remaining ingredients to heat before serving."

Preparation Time: 45 minutes

Cooking Time: Total 30 minutes

4 servings

2	pounds chicken breasts
¼	cup flour
	Salt and pepper to taste
½	pound sliced mushrooms
6	tablespoons butter, divided
2	lemons, squeezed (juice not to exceed 4 to 6 tablespoons)
½	cup chicken broth
¼	cup Marsala wine

Cut chicken into bite-sized pieces. Place in plastic bag with flour, salt, pepper and shake to coat chicken. Sauté mushrooms in 3 tablespoons butter and remove to dish, then add lemon juice. Add remaining butter to pan and cook chicken, then remove to other dish. To pan, add chicken broth and wine. Simmer 5 minutes, then add mushrooms and chicken and cook 5 to 10 minutes until hot and bubbly. Serve with rice.

Kathy Walsh
Cape Elizabeth, Maine

Tester's Note: Adding onions, garlic or parsley might enhance this already tasty dish.

chicken Reuben

"Talk about easy! I keep ingredients on hand in case of unexpected guests."

Preparation Time: 10 minutes

Baking Time: 30 minutes

6 to 8 servings

6   boneless, skinless chicken breast halves
1   15-ounce can well-drained sauerkraut
6   individual 4 x 6-inch slices Swiss cheese
1   16-ounce jar Thousand Island salad dressing

Preheat oven to 325°. Place chicken breasts in single layer in a 9 x 13-inch pan. Spoon sauerkraut over chicken. Place cheese on top of sauerkraut. Pour dressing evenly over top and bake for 30 minutes.

Marlene Duncan
Augusta, Maine

Tester's Note: This is a great recipe for sauerkraut lovers. Try it with corned beef, instead of chicken, as a variation.

chicken with Dried Fruit and wild Rice

"This is an easy, elegant dish that is wonderful for dinner parties. This recipe was given to me by a great hostess in Washington, D.C."

Preparation Time: 30 minutes

Baking Time: 1 hour

8 servings

¾	cup boiling water
2	packages onion soup
1¼	bottles Russian dressing
20	ounces apricot jam
2	pounds chicken breasts, cut in pieces
½	teaspoon minced garlic
½	teaspoon oregano
½	teaspoon curry powder
½	teaspoon poultry seasoning
	Salt to taste
2	boxes long grain and wild rice, cooked
1-1½	cups dried fruit

Preheat oven 350°. Dissolve soup in boiling water. Add Russian dressing and apricot jam. Season chicken with garlic, oregano, curry, poultry seasoning and salt. Pour soup mixture over chicken. Stir in wild rice. Add dried fruit and bake for 1 hour.

Sheila Levine
Alexandria, Virginia

chicken curry

Preparation Time: 40 to 45 minutes

Baking Time: 1 hour

6 servings

1½ cups uncooked basmati rice
2   teaspoons grated lemon peel
¼   cup raisins
6   skinned chicken breasts
    Salt and pepper to taste
2   tablespoons vegetable oil
1   onion, chopped
2   cloves garlic, minced
3   tablespoons curry powder
2   cups chicken broth
1   cup heavy cream

Preheat oven to 350°. Place rice in large, shallow baking dish. Stir in lemon peel and raisins. Arrange chicken, in one layer on top of rice. Sprinkle with salt and pepper. Heat oil in large skillet. Sauté onion and garlic until soft. Stir in curry powder and cook 2 minutes more. Stir in chicken broth and cream and bring to a slight boil. Pour over chicken. Cover tightly and bake for 1 hour, or until chicken and rice are tender.

Tall Pines Rehabilitation and Living Center
Belfast, Maine

Tester's Note: To add color interest to this recipe, try browning chicken; then toss fresh parsley on top before serving.

Creamy Baked Chicken Breasts

*"A dish so good you mustn't tell how quick and easy it is!
The recipe came from a favorite cousin and is a favorite of
all our family."*

Preparation Time: 20 minutes

Baking Time: 50 to 60 minutes

6 to 8 servings

4	whole chicken breasts, boned and skinned
8	slices of Swiss cheese
1	10¾-ounce can cream of chicken soup
¼	cup dry white wine
¼	cup orange juice
1	cup seasoned stuffing, crushed
¼	cup melted butter

Preheat oven to 350°. Arrange chicken in lightly greased baking
pan. Top with cheese slices. Combine soup, wine, and juice and
stir well. Pour over chicken evenly. Sprinkle with stuffing crumbs.
Drizzle butter over crumbs and bake for 50 to 60 minutes.

*Polly Wright
Mendon, Vermont*

Lemon Chicken

"This recipe was taught to me by my Moroccan-born husband. It has become my favorite meal, as well as a huge hit in our restaurant. It is so easy and so good! For a change, substitute salmon steaks for the chicken."

Preparation Time: 20 minutes

Cooking Time: 1hour and 30 minutes

4 servings

4   chicken legs, skinned and cut in half (8 pieces)
2   lemons, peeled and sliced
1   head of garlic, cloves peeled (use as much as desired)
½   bunch Italian parsley, chopped
1   tablespoon paprika
     Salt and pepper to taste
     Water

[handwritten note: Well, v. gd and do it's Nice to because ahead — next time, less water so broth is Thicker Oct '17 '19]

Place chicken legs in large frying pan. Place 1 slice of lemon on each piece of chicken. Place garlic around pan. Sprinkle parsley over chicken. Sprinkle paprika, salt and pepper over everything. Pour in enough water to barely cover chicken. Bring to a boil, then reduce flame and cook about 1½ hours. If too much water remains, uncover pot and let water cook down a bit. Leave enough liquid to be a "gravy". Serve with mashed potatoes (put "gravy" on potatoes), vegetable and salad.

Dorothy Almog
Santa Monica, California

Mexican Chicken

"This recipe was given to me by a lovely Mexican woman who brought it to our family after I returned from the hospital with my youngest son. My oldest son considers this his very favorite meal when he comes home to visit."

Preparation Time: 30 to 45 minutes

6 servings

4	eggs
1	bottle green chile salsa (or 2 cups homemade), divided
2	cups fine dry bread crumbs
¼	teaspoon salt
2	teaspoons each of chile powder and cumin
1½	teaspoons garlic salt
½	teaspoon oregano
6	boneless, skinless chicken breasts
¼	cup butter or olive oil
4	cups shredded lettuce
2	bunches scallions, sliced
3	tomatoes, sliced
3	limes, sliced
3	avocados, sliced

Mix eggs and half of salsa in medium bowl. Mix bread crumbs and seasonings together in another bowl. Dip chicken in salsa mixture, then bread crumb mixture. Fry slowly until done. Create each serving by laying a piece of chicken on a bed of lettuce. Then place a little salsa on chicken, followed by a dollop of sour cream on top of the salsa. Sprinkle with scallions. Garnish with tomatoes, lime and avocado.

Barbara Berv
Denver, Colorado

Staten Island Chicken

*"My mother came from Hungary; she was a wonderful cook.
I can't ever remember her using a cookbook. When she gave me
this recipe, she was living in Staten Island at the time. I have
an identical recipe, which she gave me at another time, called
"Hungarian Chicken Stew". So, call it whatever you'd like, it'll
still have an Old World taste called 'wonderful'."*

Preparation Time: 45 minutes

Cooking Time: approximately 35 minutes

6 servings

8	chicken legs, skinned
1	tablespoon grated gingerroot (or ½ tablespoon powdered ginger)
1	tablespoon vegetable or celery salt
½	tablespoon paprika
1-2	tablespoons canola oil
1	whole head of garlic, peeled and chopped
1	cup chopped parsley
5	tablespoons cornstarch
½	cup cold water
½	lemon

Spread chicken legs with mixture of ginger, salt and paprika.
Let stand for 15 to 25 minutes. Cover bottom of pot with oil,
put in garlic, parsley and seasoned chicken. Sauté, turning several
times. Then cover with boiling water (to cover half the chicken).
Cook 35 minutes. Add 5 tablespoons of cornstarch blended with
cold water. Cook, stirring, until sauce thickens. Add juice of
½ lemon.

Violet Dattner
Fresno, California

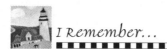

Tarragon Cream Chicken

Preparation Time: 25 minutes

Cooking Time: 10 to 15 minutes

6 servings

1   cup cream (light or heavy)
½   stick unsalted butter
4   boneless, skinless chicken breasts cut into strips or chunks
1   tablespoon dried, or ½ cup fresh tarragon, chopped
     Salt and pepper to taste
     Dash of fresh lemon juice

Heat cream and butter until thickened. Add chicken and cook until tender (only a few minutes). Add tarragon, lemon juice and salt and pepper to taste. Serve over linguine or white rice.

Carol Rodgers
Wilmington, Vermont

west Indian chicken

"This recipe is originally from Philip Anthony of Parhamtown on the island of Antigua. He cooked for my grandmother, Jean Leslie, and this was one of her favorite dishes when she lived there."

Preparation Time: 20 minutes

Baking Time: 30 to 45 minutes

6 servings

2	pounds chicken parts
2	tablespoons red wine vinegar
	Salt and pepper to taste
6	tablespoons oil
1½	tablespoons butter
2	medium onions, chopped
2	sprigs of celery, chopped
3	cloves of garlic, minced
1	green pepper, chopped
2-3	ripe tomatoes, chopped (or 1 medium can diced tomatoes)
2	tablespoons tomato paste
½ -1	cup water
	Seasoned salt (optional)

Preheat oven to 350°. Remove skin from chicken and discard. Wash chicken. Marinate chicken in vinegar, salt, pepper and oil at least 2 hours. Slightly brown chicken in butter in frying pan. Place in Dutch oven type pot with rest of ingredients. Season with salt, pepper and seasoning salt, if desired. Cook on top of stove at medium low heat or in oven for 35 to 40 minutes. Serve with rice and green salad.

Elizabeth Hatcher
Boulder, Colorado

Three Cheese Chicken Breasts in Tomato Sauce

Preparation Time: 30 minutes

Baking Time: 20 to 25 minutes

6 servings

¼	cup olive oil
6	skinless, boneless chicken breast halves
½-1	large onion, chopped
2	large cloves garlic, chopped
1	tablespoon dried oregano
1	15-ounce can tomato sauce
1	14½-ounce can Italian-style stewed tomatoes
⅓	cup dry white wine
2	bay leaves
8	ounces penne, freshly cooked
1	cup grated mozzarella cheese
⅓	cup grated Asiago or Romano cheese
⅓	cup grated Parmesan cheese

Preheat oven to 375°. Butter a 13 x 9 x 2-inch baking dish. Heat oil over high heat in large skillet. Season chicken with salt and pepper. Add chicken to skillet and sauté 1 or 2 minutes per side. Transfer to plate. Add onion, garlic and oregano to skillet and sauté until onion begins to soften, about 4 minutes. Add tomato sauce, stewed tomatoes with their juices, wine and bay leaves and cook until sauce thickens, breaking up tomatoes, about 10 minutes. Line prepared dish with penne. Arrange chicken over pasta. Spoon sauce over, covering pasta and chicken completely. Mix cheeses in small bowl. Sprinkle cheeses over sauce. Bake 20 to 25 minutes, until bubbly.

Sally Sewall
South Portland, Maine

chicken with veggies on pasta

"This is a recipe that I make whenever I am totally bored with the 'usual' meals or I have a great need for veggies. It's easy, not too messy, and provides a complete meal for a dinner. It can also be made with just veggies, or with shrimp instead of chicken."

Preparation Time: 30 minutes

4 to 6 servings

1   pound chicken breasts
1-2 tablespoons olive oil
1   pound linguine, or favorite pasta
½   green pepper, cut into inch pieces
½   red or yellow pepper, cut into inch pieces
2   celery stalks, sliced into ¼-inch thickness
1   small onion, diced
3   large mushrooms, diced
1   teaspoon roasted garlic
1   can chopped tomatoes with garlic and olive oil
½   teaspoon oregano
½   teaspoon basil
     Salt and pepper to taste

Cut chicken breast into 1-inch chunks. Sauté in olive oil. Cook pasta as instructed on package. In a non-stick skillet, add remaining ingredients. Sauté on medium heat for 7 minutes. Reduce heat to simmer and cover until done. Drain pasta, put on plates, add veggies and chicken. Enjoy with your favorite bread and red wine.

Larry Braziel
Cape Elizabeth, Maine

Hot Turkey Salad

"This was the traditional day after Thanksgiving meal that my mother always made. An excellent way to use up that leftover turkey! It is excellent as a cold salad as well. It provides a nice combination of crunchy and soft."

Preparation Time: 20 minutes

Baking Time: 15 minutes, or until heated through

4 servings

2	cups cooked turkey, cut into bite-sized pieces
2	cups chopped celery
¼	cup chopped nuts (optional)
1	tablespoon lemon juice
	Pinch of salt
2	heaping tablespoons of mayonnaise
	Potato chips
⅓	cup grated cheddar cheese

Preheat oven to 450°. Mix turkey, celery, nuts, lemon juice and salt together. Add enough mayonnaise to moisten it all. Spoon into casserole dish. Top with crushed potato chips and sprinkle with grated cheddar cheese. (Corn flakes can be substituted for potato chips). Bake for 15 minutes or until heated through. Serve warm.

Jim Donahue
Cumberland, Maine

Turkey Breast

Preparation Time: 15 to 20 minutes

Baking Time: 20 minutes per pound

8 to 10 servings

1   whole turkey breast (approximately 4½ pounds)
3   good-sized shallots
½   cup chicken broth
½   cup dry vermouth
     Oil, canola or olive
     Paprika
     Salt and pepper

Preheat oven to 325°. Cut fat from turkey breast and discard. Rinse turkey in cold water, dry and rub oil over skin then sprinkle with paprika, salt and pepper. Chop up shallots. Put breast in roasting pan, after rubbing bottom of pan with oil. Sprinkle shallots around breast, pour broth and vermouth into pan. Roast 20 minutes per pound. Check for doneness, as oven temperatures vary.

Barbara Pratt
Scarborough, Maine

Tester's Note: This is a very easy recipe that smells wonderful when cooking and makes a very flavorful sauce.

candied cornish Game Hens

"This recipe is almost as good without the chutney. A favorite around Christmas time when everyone is tired of turkey. It is simple to do."

Preparation Time: approximately 1 hour

Baking Time: 1 hour

4 servings

4	Cornish game hens, 1¼ to 1½ pounds each
	Salt, pepper and poultry seasoning
⅓	cup melted butter
⅓	cup honey
⅓	cup granulated sugar
2	teaspoons cinnamon

Preheat oven to 350°. Remove giblets, wash hens and season inside of cavity with salt and pepper and a little poultry seasoning. Place in baking pan. Cover loosely with foil and bake 30 minutes. Remove from oven and raise temperature to 400°. Whisk together butter and honey and brush it generously on hens, coating the whole bird. Mix cinnamon and sugar, sprinkle over birds and bake, uncovered an additional 30 minutes. The hens are done when juices run clear, not pink, or meat thermometer inserted midway between thigh and breast reaches 180°. Serve with Cranberry Chutney (recipe follows).

Paul Miller, Chef of The Cornish Inn
Cornish, Maine

cranberry chutney

"This is much better with poultry than ordinary cranberry sauce."

Preparation Time: 20 minutes

Cooking Time: 1 hour 10 minutes

4 to 6 servings

1	cup quartered and sliced onions
1	cup water
¾	cup dark brown sugar
½	cup granulated sugar
¾	cup cider vinegar
2-3	Granny Smith apples cored, peeled and diced
½	teaspoon salt
1	teaspoon grated, fresh ginger
½	teaspoon mace
¼	teaspoon ground cloves
½	teaspoon curry powder
	Zest of two oranges, grated fine
1	quart cranberries
½	cup currants
	Juice of two oranges

Combine first 4 ingredients in a heavy saucepan and simmer 30 minutes. Add next 8 ingredients, bring to a slow boil and cook 30 minutes. Add last three ingredients and continue to boil slowly for 10 minutes, or until cranberries burst. Serve warm or at room temperature with Cornish game hens, or most any poultry.

Paul Miller, Chef of The Cornish Inn
Cornish, Maine

Tester's Note: This recipe is time-consuming, but very tasty. Perhaps it would be a good idea to make it ahead of time.

Baked Stuffed Scallops

"An easy recipe that looks like you worked for hours. Stuffing can be used with other seafood too."

Preparation Time: 20 minutes

Baking Time: 30 minutes

4 servings

2	cups Italian-style bread crumbs
½	cup butter, melted
6	ounces baby shrimp, canned or fresh
2	tablespoons lemon juice
1½-2	pounds bay scallops, fresh or frozen and thawed

Preheat oven to 350°. Pour bread crumbs, butter, shrimp and lemon juice into small bowl and mix well. Mixture should be completely moist and clump well. Sprinkle 1 to 2 tablespoons of stuffing into 8x8-inch or 9x9-inch baking pan. Add scallops and top with remaining stuffing. Scallops should be no more than 2 layers deep. Stuffing should pack in nicely and just coat the top. Bake for approximately 30 minutes or until scallops are white.

Karen Byram
Scarborough, Maine

Molasses Marinated Scallops

Preparation Time: 15 minutes

1 serving

½ cup molasses
½ cup brewed coffee
4 large scallops

Chutney
2 tablespoons diced onion
½ cup pineapple, diced
2 tablespoons vinegar
1 tablespoon sugar
½ tablespoon curry powder
1-2 tablespoons vegetable oil

Mix molasses and coffee and marinate scallops in mixture for at least 5 minutes. Sauté onions and pineapple; add vinegar, sugar and curry powder. Boil for a few minutes to reduce liquid. Sear scallops in oil on both sides and serve over chutney.

William Boutwell, BiBo's Madd Apple Café
Portland, Maine

Soy-Glazed Salmon

"I started to make this recipe a few years ago when we were told how good salmon is for us. It is high in protein and low in fat. This is a great recipe for your friends that do not eat red meat. My guests always think I went overboard to fix this winner."

Preparation Time: 10 minutes

4 servings

3	tablespoons reduced-sodium soy sauce
1½	tablespoons orange juice
1½	tablespoons honey
1	tablespoon grated fresh ginger
⅛	teaspoon hot red pepper flakes
4	6-ounce salmon steaks, ¾-inch thick
	Cooking spray

In a small bowl mix first 5 ingredients. Pour all but 1 tablespoon into large, plastic, resealable food storage bag. Add salmon steaks, seal and turn to coat. Let salmon marinate 5 to 10 minutes. Preheat broiler. Lightly coat broiler pan with cooking spray. Remove salmon from bag and arrange on broiler pan. Reserve marinade in bag. Broil salmon steaks 4 minutes, turn over; brush with marinade from the bag and broil 3 to 5 minutes until opaque at center. Transfer to plates, top with reserved 1 tablespoon of marinade and serve.

SuSu DePaolo
South Portland, Maine

Poached Salmon

"I've never served this without rave reviews."

Preparation Time: 15 minutes

4 servings

1½ pounds salmon
    Juice of one lemon
    Salt to taste
    Dried dill

Preheat oven to 375°. Put a piece of foil large enough to wrap salmon in a shallow baking dish. Place salmon on top of foil. Spread lemon juice on top of salmon. Sprinkle lightly with salt. Add dill generously to lightly cover salmon. Wrap foil around salmon and seal to make airtight. Bake for 5 minutes per inch width of salmon.

Barbara Nelson
Littleton, Colorado

Barbeque Roasted Salmon

"My sister is the best cook I know. She periodically gives me recipes that are simple yet elegant. This one fits that bill, especially for salmon lovers. Don't let the name of the recipe fool you. It's actually baked, not barbecued."

Preparation Time: 15 minutes

Baking Time: 20 to 30 minutes

4 servings

4	6-ounce salmon fillets
¼	cup pineapple juice
2	tablespoons fresh lemon juice
2	tablespoons brown sugar
2-4	teaspoons chili powder
2	teaspoons grated lemon rind
¾	teaspoon ground cumin
½	teaspoon salt
¼	teaspoon cinnamon
	Lemon wedges

Preheat oven to 350°. Rinse salmon under cold water and lay skin-side down in 9x13-inch baking pan. Mix pineapple juice and lemon juice together and pour over salmon. Let stand 1 hour. Combine brown sugar, chili powder, lemon rind, cumin, salt and cinnamon. Spoon mixture over salmon. Bake for 20 to 30 minutes, depending on thickness of salmon. Serve with lemon wedges.

Katherine Beach
South Portland, Maine

Baked Salmon Fillets

"This is good hot or cold. My son-in-law brought the recipe from Chicago to Bath. It is wonderfully simple for entertaining."

Preparation Time: 5 minutes

Baking Time: 20 minutes

3 servings

1	pound salmon fillets
½	cup Scotch or Bourbon whiskey
½	cup olive oil
¼	cup soy sauce

Preheat oven to 400°. Line baking dish with foil and place salmon in dish. Mix together whiskey, olive oil and soy sauce. Pour over salmon. Let salmon marinate for awhile in the refrigerator. (Length of time not too important). Bake for 20 minutes. Do not overcook.

Ada Recknagel
Bath, Maine

Tester's Note: Watch carefully when baking, as marinade may flame briefly. You may pour off most of the marinade before baking to avoid this problem. Tastes great!!

Salmon Loaf

"My mother used to run a boarding house and this was one of the favorites."

Preparation Time: 30 minutes

Baking Time: 40 to 50 minutes

4 to 6 servings

1   14¾-ounce can salmon
1   egg
1   small onion, finely chopped
¼   cup finely chopped green pepper
½   cup mashed potato
¼   cup milk
     Salt and pepper, to taste

White Sauce
1   tablespoon butter
1   tablespoon flour
1   cup milk
2   hard-boiled eggs, chopped
1   8½-ounce can peas
     Salt and pepper to taste

Preheat oven to 325°. Mix salmon, egg, onion, pepper, potato, milk, salt and pepper. Place in greased loaf pan and bake for 40 to 50 minutes. For white sauce, melt butter in saucepan and stir in flour. Gradually add milk and stir until thickened. Add hard-boiled eggs and peas. Serve sauce over salmon loaf.

Sheryl Waisanen
West Paris, Maine

Very good!
Nov '10

Baked Fish

"This recipe came from Central Maine Power Company years ago when they sent out recipes with their bills."

Preparation Time: 15 minutes

Baking Time: 20 minutes

4 servings

1½ pounds white fish fillets (sole, haddock, etc.)
1   cup dairy sour cream
1   teaspoon lemon juice
½   teaspoon salt
1   teaspoon honey
2   tablespoons fine bread crumbs
    Paprika

Preheat oven to 400°. Arrange fillets in greased baking pan. Mix together sour cream, lemon juice, salt, honey and bread crumbs. Spread over fish. Bake for 20 minutes or until fish flakes with fork and topping is lightly brown. Remove from oven; sprinkle with paprika and serve.

Fran Johnson
Las Cruces, New Mexico

New England Cod Cakes

Preparation Time: 25 minutes

10 cakes

1   pound cod fillets, skinless and boneless
½   cup mayonnaise
¼   cup finely chopped chives
     Salt and pepper to taste
     Fresh ground white bread crumbs
3   ounces butter

Cut cod into 2x2-inch pieces and steam until ¾ done. Cool in strainer to drain juices. In bowl fold together cod, mayonnaise, chives, salt and pepper. Scoop into 2 ounce balls on a bread crumb dusted table and carefully form into cakes using bread crumbs as needed (do not overwork or incorporate excessive bread crumbs). Heat sauce pan, add butter and when sizzles, sauté cakes until golden brown on both sides. Serve with salad and tomato tartar sauce or as an appetizer.

Executive Chef Daniel Bruce
Boston Harbor Hotel Boston, Massachusetts

Best if served with sauce for added flavor.

Haddock casserole

"This tasty recipe became a favorite of my mom's and she served it often to family and friends invited to dinner. Mom would also serve her famous tossed green salad with Italian dressing and rolls with this meal."

Preparation Time: 20 minutes

Baking Time: 30 to 40 minutes

4 to 5 servings

1½-2	pounds haddock
¼	cup chopped onion
2	tablespoons butter or margarine
2	tablespoons flour
¼	teaspoon salt
⅛	teaspoon pepper
1	cup milk
1	cup cheddar cheese, shredded
1	cup sour cream
1	10-ounce can mushroom soup
1	cup frozen peas, thawed
	Crushed crackers (optional)

Preheat oven to 350°. Put fish in 9x13-inch baking pan.
Sauté onion in butter until soft. Add flour, salt and pepper and stir until mixed. Add milk to mixture and stir over medium heat until smooth and creamy. Add cheddar cheese; stir until melted. Mix in sour cream, mushroom soup (undiluted) and peas.
Stir sauce until well mixed. Pour over fish. Sprinkle with crushed crackers (if desired). Bake 30 to 40 minutes. This recipe may be put together early in the day and refrigerated until cooking time.

Elizabeth McLeod
South Portland, Maine

Grilled Salmon with Peach Bourbon Barbecue Sauce

Preparation Time: 45 to 55 minutes

8 servings

Barbecue Sauce
3   tablespoons Worcestershire sauce
3   tablespoons soy sauce
¾   teaspoon allspice
¾   teaspoon chili powder
¾   teaspoon dried basil
¾   teaspoon ground oregano
¾   teaspoon minced ginger root
¾   teaspoon black pepper
1½   teaspoons dry mustard
¼   cup plus 2 teaspoons cider vinegar
¾   teaspoon celery seeds
1   15-ounce can peaches, drained
1⅓   cups basic barbecue sauce (homemade is best)
1½   tablespoons butter, melted
½   cup plus 2 tablespoons lemon juice
⅛   teaspoon liquid smoke flavoring
½   cup brown sugar
⅓   cup catsup
3   tablespoons pineapple juice
3   tablespoons bourbon

Salmon
4   pounds salmon fillets, skinned and boned
½   cup olive oil
2   tablespoon minced garlic
1   teaspoon salt
1   teaspoon pepper

At least one day before serving, prepare barbecue sauce. Process first 11 ingredients in blender to incorporate dry seasonings. Pour into large bowl or jar. Process peaches in blender; add ¾ cup peach purée and remaining sauce ingredients to bowl. Mix well and refrigerate overnight. Two hours before cooking, cut salmon into 8 equal pieces. Place in dish to marinate with garlic, oil, salt and pepper. When ready to cook, preheat grill and put sauce in pan to warm slowly. Cook fillets on grill about 3 minutes. Turn and cook for 2 to 3 minutes more, or until fish begins to flake when tested with fork. Fish is best when slightly undercooked. Place piece of salmon on each of 8 plates. Ladle ¼ cup warmed sauce in pool beside each serving.

The Island Inn (Chef: Duane Judson)
Monhegan Island, Maine

Note: We serve this with red beans and rice and Asian vegetables (bok choy, napa cabbage, bean sprouts, scallions) sautéed with garlic and sesame oil. Leftover sauce may be refrigerated for at least a week or frozen to use at a later date. Sauce recipe may also be halved.

Baked Fish à la Ritz

Preparation Time: 15 minutes

Baking Time: 30 to 35 minutes

6 to 8 servings

2   pounds pollock or haddock fillets
¼   pound Ritz crackers, cheese or plain, crumbled
2   tablespoons Parmesan cheese
⅓   cup 2% milk

Preheat oven to 325°. Place fish in buttered 9x13x2-inch baking pan. Combine crackers and cheese, in food processor. Process mixture into crumbs. Put crumbs in bowl, add milk and mix. Spread crumbs on fish. Bake for 30 to 35 minutes, or until fish is flaky.

The Lamp, Alzheimer's Residential Care Facility
Lisbon, Maine

Clam Fritters

"When we were kids, we loved digging for clams. Mom liked to come along for the dig, but not being much of a cook, she got her friend, Alice, to make these fritters for us."

Preparation Time: 20 minutes

4 servings

1   pint shucked and chopped steamers (Maine soft shell clams)
1½ cups cracker crumbs (use crackers with salted tops)
2   tablespoons finely minced onion
2   eggs
    Salt and pepper
    Vegetable oil for frying

Mix clams, crumbs and onion together. Add eggs, one at a time, mixing well. Stir in salt and pepper to taste. Let mixture stand a few minutes to soften crumbs. Heat 2 or 3 tablespoons of vegetable oil in sauté pan over medium heat. Drop mixture in large spoonfuls into hot pan, flattening to make fritters about ¾-inch thick. Cook until golden on both sides. Serve with tartar sauce.

Sally Sewall
South Portland, Maine

Soused Steamers

"Summers in Maine, with all generations of our family together, we have a rule: Everyone either cooks or cleans up. This recipe evolved over many happy evenings with too many cooks in the kitchen."

Preparation Time: ½ hour

Cooking Time: 5 to 10 minutes

8 servings as appetizer, 4 servings as entrée

8   dozen steamers, soaked for an hour in salt water with
      ½ cup vinegar added to purge sand, then rinsed
½   cup water
1   cup (or more) dry white wine
2-3 cloves garlic, sliced
1   medium onion, sliced
½   teaspoon dried tarragon
½   teaspoon salt
2   tablespoons butter
8   whole peppercorns
1   stick butter, melted (for dipping)

Combine water, wine, onion, garlic, tarragon, salt, 2 tablespoons butter and peppercorns in a large pot. Bring all to boil and simmer for 5 minutes. Add clams to pot, cover and steam until all the clams are open, about 5 to 10 minutes. Discard broken clams or those that don't open. Remove clams to serving bowl. Pour broth into mugs and melted butter into little bowls for each person. Drink the broth and eat the onions when the clams are gone.

Patricia Noonan
Purchase, New York

crab cakes

"These also make wonderful appetizers. Just make small bite-size cakes and cook the same way. Great for party."

Preparation Time: 15 to 20 minutes

6 cakes

1	pound crabmeat
2	eggs, beaten
2	tablespoons butter or margarine, melted
2	tablespoons salad dressing or mayonnaise
1	teaspoon salt
¼	teaspoon ginger
1	teaspoon dried parsley flakes
½	teaspoon dry mustard
1	teaspoon Worcestershire sauce
	Cream, enough to hold mixture together (if necessary)
1	cup bread crumbs

Combine all above ingredients except bread crumbs. Form cakes and roll in bread crumbs. Fry in skillet or deep fryer.

Peg Furey
Falmouth, Maine

crab Baltimore

"This is a recipe that reminds me of my mom and summer. She loved serving this on a hot summer night. It comes all the way from Baltimore, Maryland where she lived during the war and where I was born. It has been with me a long time and never gets old."

Preparation Time: 20 minutes

Baking Time: 15 minutes

4 servings as entrée, 8 servings as appetizer

1	pound crabmeat
½	green pepper, minced
½	pimiento, minced
1	tablespoon lemon juice
1	teaspoon Worcestershire sauce
½	cup mayonnaise
3	drops Tabasco sauce
½	teaspoon dry mustard
¼	teaspoon salt
¼	teaspoon white pepper
4	tablespoons bread crumbs
2	tablespoons butter

Preheat oven to 375°. Combine all ingredients except bread crumbs and butter. Combine bread crumbs and butter with fingers. Put mixture in a buttered casserole dish and top with bread crumb mixture. Bake on a baking sheet for 15 minutes. (For appetizer servings bake in scallop shells or ramekins.)

Peggy Greenhut Golden
Cumberland Foreside, Maine

Spicy Shrimp Curry

"Excellent served with basmati rice or stuffed potato breads."

Preparation Time: 1 hour

4 servings

3	tablespoons butter or oil (do not use olive oil)
1	medium onion, finely chopped
¼	teaspoon turmeric
½	tablespoon minced fresh ginger
2	small green chiles, minced
2	cloves garlic, minced
1	cup canned peeled, crushed tomatoes, chopped
1	pound shrimp, peeled and deveined
½-1	cup coconut milk
¼	teaspoon garam masala (optional) (found in Indian or Middle Eastern grocery stores)
	Salt and pepper
¼	cup chopped cilantro, stems and leaves

Heat butter or oil in a skillet on medium heat. Add onion and turmeric and cook for 10 to 15 minutes, or until onions are soft. Add ginger, chiles and garlic. Cook for 3 minutes. Turn heat up to medium high and add tomatoes; cook 5 to 10 minutes. Add shrimp and cook 3 to 5 minutes until shrimp are bright orange. Do not overcook. Turn heat down to medium and add coconut milk to desired consistency. Turn off heat and let sit for a minute. Add optional garam masala and salt and pepper to taste. Before serving stir in cilantro.

Mary Taddia
Portland, Maine

Jinnie's Stuffed Striped Bass

"This recipe takes me back more than 60 years to happy days spent surf fishing for stripers with my father on the beach at Ship's Bottom, New Jersey."

Preparation Time: 15 minutes

Baking Time: 1 hour

1   striped bass, cleaned

Stuffing
Use following ingredients in proportion to size of fish
    Soft bread crumbs
    Chopped celery
    Chopped onion
    Chopped parsley
    Salt and pepper
    Thyme
    Sage
    Melted butter

Topping
    Sliced bacon
    Sliced tomato
    Sliced onion
    White Wine
    Melted butter

Preheat oven to 350°. Take striped bass and open larger pocket in center by running a sharp knife down the backbone from the inside. Mix stuffing ingredients together and fill the pocket with stuffing. Secure with toothpicks. Wrap bass in bacon strips. Top with tomato and onion slices. Lay bass on large piece of aluminum foil and wrap bass, crimping edges of foil. Foil should not be too tight around fish. Bake for 30 minutes. Open foil wide. Baste fish with white wine and melted butter. Raise heat to 375° and bake for 30 minutes more.

Virginia M. Self
Yarmouth, Maine

Cioppino

"This recipe was shared with me for the first time back in the early 1990's at the home of Don and Jane Leeber. It is a favorite with good Tuscan bread and a green salad. Easy because most of the preparation is done the day before, leaving lots of time with your company."

Preparation Time: 1 hour

Cooking Time: 1½ hours

6 servings

Tomato Base
¼	cup olive oil
2	tablespoons butter
1	cup finely chopped onion
1	cup chopped green pepper
1	teaspoon minced garlic
1	pound fresh mushrooms, cut in half if large
1	28-ounce can crushed tomatoes with added purée and basil
1	6-ounce can tomato paste
1	cup dry white wine
2	8-ounce bottles clam juice
2	tablespoons minced fresh parsley
¼	cup fresh lemon juice
2	bay leaves
1	teaspoon dried oregano
½	teaspoon dried basil
½	teaspoon salt
½	teaspoon pepper
1	tablespoon sugar

Fish
1½	pounds swordfish, sea bass or red snapper, cut in 1-to 2-inch cubes
1	dozen mussels, cleaned
1	pound medium shrimp, peeled and deveined
½	pound scallops, rinsed clean
½	pound lump crabmeat, picked over to remove shells

For tomato base: heat oil and butter over medium heat in large Dutch oven. Add onion, green pepper, garlic and mushrooms. Cook until onions are limp, about 10 minutes. Add tomatoes, tomato paste, wine, clam juice, parsley, lemon juice, bay leaves, oregano, basil, salt, pepper and sugar. Heat to boil; reduce heat and simmer, covered, over low heat 1 hour. Refrigerate. (Can be made up to 48 hours in advance.) Half hour before serving heat tomato base to a simmer. Add cubed fish; cook until almost flaky, 10 to 15 minutes. Add mussels, shrimp, scallops and crabmeat. Cover and simmer over low heat until mussels open, about 10 minutes. Spoon into flat soup bowls and serve.

Peggy Greenhut Golden
Cumberland Foreside, Maine

Tester's Note: To garnish, if desired, mix together mayonnaise, curry powder and lime juice to taste. Put a dollop on each serving.

Swordfish à la spike

"Recipe originally came from Brighton Medical Center chef, Tom. It is great for unexpected guests, sailing weekends or at home with friends. The fish melts in your mouth."

Preparation Time: 5 minutes

8 servings

8   8-ounce pieces of swordfish
1   cup Chablis, or other dry white wine
½   cup Dijon mustard
½   cup soy sauce (reduced-sodium variety works well)
4   tablespoons honey
4   teaspoons curry powder

In a bowl, mix all ingredients except fish. Pour over fish and marinate for at least 1 hour and up to 8 hours. Grill fish 6 to 8 minutes on each side, basting with marinade.

Sandy Enck
Scarborough, Maine

Baked Scrod

"This can also be done with halibut or haddock. I like to serve white and wild rice with it."

Preparation Time: 15 minutes

Baking Time: 20 minutes

4 servings

¼ cup butter or margarine
2 large shallots or ½ cup minced onion
2 cups fresh bread crumbs
¼ cup chopped fresh chives
3 tablespoons minced fresh parsley
2 teaspoons grated lemon peel
   Salt and pepper to taste
1½ pounds scrod fillets
2 tablespoons fresh lemon juice
   Lemon wedges for garnish

Preheat oven to 450°. Melt butter, add onion and cook one minute. Add bread crumbs and stir until butter is absorbed. Remove from heat, add chives, parsley and lemon peel. Season to taste with salt and pepper. Spray baking pan with vegetable oil. Place fish in pan and brush with lemon juice. Cover with bread crumb mixture, pressing crumbs onto fish. Bake about 20 minutes. Serve with lemon wedges.

Elinor Clark
Skowhegan, Maine

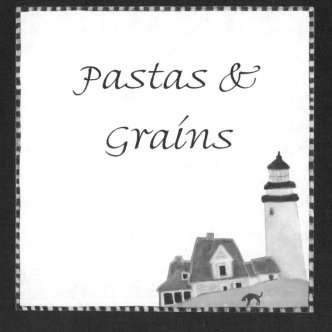

Pastas &
Grains

Old Fashioned Macaroni and Cheese

"Warning! Once you have had this macaroni and cheese, it is difficult to eat boxed macaroni and cheese ever again."

Preparation Time: 30 minutes

Baking Time: 30 minutes

4 to 6 servings

1	8-ounce box elbow macaroni
5	tablespoons butter, divided
3	tablespoons flour
1	teaspoon salt
¼	teaspoon pepper
1	teaspoon dry mustard
3	cups scalded milk
1	10-ounce package sharp cheddar cheese, cubed or grated
½	package Pepperidge Farm Stuffing, not cubed

Preheat oven to 325°. Cook macaroni according to package directions. Drain and rinse with cool water. Set aside.
Melt 3 tablespoons butter in a double boiler. Add flour, salt, pepper, and dry mustard to make a thick paste. Remove pan from heat. Add warm milk slowly, stirring constantly. Try to avoid any lumps. Return pan to heat and add cheese. Continue to stir slowly until cheese is melted and sauce starts to thicken. Put macaroni in large casserole dish and pour cheese over it. Stir gently until mixed thoroughly. Melt remaining 2 tablespoons of butter in separate dish and add stuffing mix. Mix well. Cover top of macaroni with stuffing. Bake for 30 minutes uncovered.

Lyn Donahue
Cumberland, Maine

Tester's Note: I reduced the amount of stuffing to 2 cups and the butter to 2 tablespoons.

Macaroni and Cheese Casserole

Preparation Time: ½ hour

Baking Time: 30 minutes

6 to 8 servings

2	cups macaroni
½	stick butter
2	tablespoons flour
1	teaspoon dry mustard
½	teaspoon salt
1½	cups evaporated milk
2	cups shredded cheddar cheese
1	cup diced cooked ham
1	cup cooked peas
1	cup crushed buttery crackers

Preheat oven to 350°. Cook macaroni, drain. Return to pot. Add butter, flour, dry mustard and salt, stirring constantly over medium heat until butter is melted. Stir in evaporated milk. Cook stirring constantly for 1 to 2 minutes. Add cheese. Stir until melted. Add ham and peas. Spread in 9 x 13-inch pan. Cover with cracker crumbs. Bake for 30 minutes. Serve piping hot.

Pat Cunningham
Belfast, Maine

Florida Pasta

"Before boarding the plane for our annual family April vacation in Sanibel Island, Florida during the 1980's, I would stock up on several women's magazines. I enjoyed using some time during the vacation trying out the recipes in the magazines. Working as a teacher didn't leave me much time for cooking except during vacation. This recipe was an instant hit with my family. It has become one of my favorites because of the few, simple ingredients, the ease of preparation, and the wonderful taste. We now call it Florida Pasta."

Preparation Time: 20 minutes

4 servings

¼   cup olive oil
2   cloves garlic, minced
3-4   medium ripe tomatoes, diced
8   ounces mozzarella cheese, cubed
½-¾ pound dry pasta (or ¾ to 1 pound fresh pasta)
     Black olives, halved (optional)

Heat oil over medium heat and sauté garlic until lightly browned. Set aside. Meanwhile, cook pasta as directed, drain. Return to pot. Toss pasta with remaining ingredients. Allow to sit for several minutes to infuse flavors and to slightly melt the cheese.

Carolyn Davis
Cape Elizabeth, Maine

Broccoli and Macaroni à la Barbara

"When I was a teenager, I had no desire to learn to cook. My mother, fearing I would starve to death while living off campus at college, gave me this simple, healthy recipe that my family still enjoys today!"

Preparation Time: 30 minutes

4 servings

1	head broccoli
¼	cup olive oil
2-3	cloves of garlic
1	pound pasta
½	cup grated Romano cheese
	Fresh ground pepper

Divide broccoli into florets and steam until crunchy. (Do not overcook!) Gently sauté garlic in olive oil without browning. Add broccoli and sauté until well mixed with garlic and oil, about 1 minute. Cook pasta "al dente." Drain, reserving 1 cup of water. Add broccoli mixture to pasta. Sprinkle with cheese and add pepper to taste. If dry, add some of the reserved water a little at a time. Serve with additional pepper and cheese.

Denise McLeod
Doylestown, Pennsylvania

Baked Shells with Green Sauce

"My mother had a thing about children (all six of us!) eating our spinach, so she disguised it as "green sauce" and told us that if we ever wanted to get to the moon, we'd have to eat it."

Preparation Time: 30 minutes

Baking Time: 12 minutes

6 to 8 servings

2	pounds spinach
1	stick butter, divided
1	cup chicken stock
½	teaspoon basil
¼	teaspoon garlic powder
	Salt and pepper to taste
1¼	cups Parmesan cheese
1	pound shells
8	tablespoons bread crumbs

Preheat oven to 425°. Cook spinach quickly (5 minutes), drain and chop finely. Melt 1½ tablespoons butter in saucepan. Add chopped spinach. Stir 5 minutes and add chicken stock. Boil fiercely to reduce stock for 3 to 5 minutes. Add seasonings and 1 cup cheese. Sauce will thicken. Cook pasta 5 minutes less than directions specify; drain and toss with 5 tablespoons melted butter. Butter bottom of deep oven dish and alternate layers of pasta and green sauce, ending with a pasta layer. Cover with bread crumbs and remaining cheese. Dot with remaining butter. Bake 10 minutes Place under broiler for 2 minutes or until top is lightly browned.

Pat Lambrew
Scarborough, Maine

Sesame Peanut Noodles

"This foolproof recipe was given to me by a friend in Portsmouth, NH. I've made it countless times. It is always popular at parties, potlucks, picnics and family dinners. If you prefer dishes that are not too spicy, cut back on the salt and garlic and use only 2 tablespoons of hot oil."

Preparation Time: 20 to 25 minutes

4 to 5 servings

4   cloves garlic, minced
2-4 tablespoons hot oil (available in the Chinese food section.)
4   tablespoons sesame oil
4   tablespoons peanut butter (smooth or crunchy)
5-6 tablespoons warm water
2   teaspoons salt
3-4 tablespoons sugar
4   tablespoons Tamari sauce
2   tablespoons wine vinegar
1   pound soft Chinese-style noodles (available in natural food
        refrigerator section)
4   tablespoons minced scallions

In a measuring cup, mix together all ingredients except noodles and scallions. Boil noodles according to package directions, making sure not to overcook. Pour cooked, drained noodles into large bowl. Add sauce and mix well. Garnish with minced scallions. Serve immediately, or chill and serve later.

Elizabeth Lantz
Portland, Maine

Linguine with Clam Sauce

"This recipe was given to me by my mother. It is wonderful on a cold, winter day!"

Preparation Time: 20 to 25 minutes

4 servings

8	ounces linguine
8	ounces clam juice
⅛	cup olive oil
1	tablespoon vinegar
1	envelope garlic/herb salad dressing
3	dozen clams, shucked or 1 pound minced clams
1	tablespoon parsley
2	tablespoons basil

Cook linguine until desired tenderness. Bring clam juice, oil, vinegar and salad dressing mix to a boil. Add clams. Reduce heat to low. Simmer for 5 minutes. Stir in parsley and basil. Pour over linguine. Serve immediately.

Christy Peters
Augusta, Maine

Tester's Note: I would suggest using fresh parsley and basil, especially since the recipe calls for prepared salad dressing.

Shrimp Fettuccine

Preparation Time: 20 minutes

4 servings

1   pound fresh or frozen shrimp, cooked, peeled and deveined
1   4-ounce can mushroom stems and pieces, drained
½   teaspoon garlic powder
⅛   teaspoon salt
⅛   teaspoon pepper
¼   cup margarine
1   8-ounce package fettuccine, cooked and drained
½   cup grated Parmesan cheese
½   cup milk
½   cup sour cream
½   tablespoon dried parsley

In a large saucepan, sauté shrimp, mushrooms, garlic powder, salt and pepper in margarine for 3 to 5 minutes. Stir in fettuccine, cheese, milk, sour cream, and parsley flakes. Cook over medium heat for 3 to 5 minutes or until heated through. Do not boil.

Carol Furlong
Eagle Lake, Maine

Note: Scallops or lobster may be substituted for half the shrimp.

Pasta with Tomato-Crabmeat Sauce

"This is an attempt to duplicate a memorable meal that my husband and I had in Corniglia, one of the villages of the Cinque Terre, in Italy. The village is high on a cliff overlooking the Ligurian Sea and only accessible by train. The restaurant, called Cecios, was run by one family. The mother, who did all of the cooking, yelled orders from the kitchen in Italian. Her son, our waiter, was the only one in the village who spoke English. Their version of the pasta had a nice crabmeat flavor, but no discernible chunks of crab. Enjoy!"

Preparation Time: 20 minutes

4 to 6 servings

2-3	tablespoons olive oil
8	cloves garlic, minced
½	teaspoon crushed red pepper
1	28-ounce can crushed tomatoes in purée
	Pinch of salt
6	ounces fresh crabmeat
1	pound pasta (ziti or penne)
2	tablespoons vodka
½	cup heavy cream
¼	cup chopped parsley

Combine olive oil, garlic and crushed red pepper in large skillet. Cook over moderate heat until garlic turns golden brown. Add canned tomatoes and a pinch of salt. Stir, simmer uncovered about 15 minutes. Add crabmeat. Keep warm. Cook pasta "al dente." Add drained pasta to tomato sauce and mix well. Add vodka, mix; add cream, mix again. Cover, reduce heat to low and simmer for 1 to 2 minutes. Add parsley. Serve in warmed pasta bowls.

Nancy Lombardelli
South Portland, Maine

Noodles Delight

Preparation Time: 10 to 15 minutes

6 servings

3   packages chicken Oodles of Noodles
2   tablespoons margarine
1   10-ounce package frozen mixed vegetables, thawed and
      drained
1   10¾-ounce can cream of asparagus soup
¾   cup milk
1½ cups shredded mozzarella cheese
1   7-ounce can tuna, drained

Cook noodles according to the package directions. Add seasoning
packets. Drain off most of the liquid. Set aside. In large skillet
cook vegetables in margarine over medium heat, 2 minutes;
stirring often. Stir in the asparagus soup and milk. Add cheese.
Cook until cheese melts, stirring occasionally. Stir in noodles and
tuna. Heat through, stirring often.

Gerri Reny
South Portland, Maine

Note: You can use any vegetable you like in place of the mixed
vegetables or use salmon instead of tuna.

Energizing Linguine

"Great dish for weight watchers that the whole family will enjoy. Easy to prepare and very filling. Can use leftover turkey or chicken."

Preparation Time: 45 minutes

4 servings

8	ounces linguine
1	tablespoon butter or margarine
1	cup sliced fresh mushrooms
½	cup sliced celery
2	tablespoons cornstarch
½	cup dry white wine
1	cup chicken broth
2	teaspoons lemon juice
¼	teaspoon dried thyme, crushed
2-3	dashes hot pepper sauce
½	cup shredded mozzarella cheese
1½	cups cooked chicken or turkey cut in strips
4	ounces fresh spinach, chopped
	Grated Parmesan cheese (optional)

Prepare linguine according to package directions, omitting salt. Drain and keep warm. Melt butter or margarine in medium saucepan. Add mushrooms and celery. Stir in cornstarch. Cook until tender. Add next 5 ingredients and stir until bubbly. Stir in cheese until melted. Add chicken or turkey and spinach. Cover and cook 1 minute or until heated through. Pour over warm linguine. You may then sprinkle with Parmesan cheese if you like.

Sandy Enck
Scarborough, Maine

Pasta Carbonara

Preparation Time: ½ hour

6 to 8 servings

¼   pound bacon, cut into small pieces
2   tablespoons butter
1   cup milk
2   tablespoons wine vinegar
2   eggs, beaten
1   pound favorite pasta
⅓   cup Parmesan or Romano cheese, freshly grated
     Salt and pepper to taste

Cook the bacon in butter until bacon is transparent. Heat the milk in a small saucepan and add bacon and butter. Add wine vinegar to mixture. (This will turn the milk to cheese.) Simmer for about 15 minutes or until smooth. Cook pasta in salted water, drain and return to pot. Immediately add 2 beaten eggs, sauce, grated cheese, salt and pepper to pasta. Toss well and serve hot.

The Honorable John E. Baldacci, U.S. Congressman
Bangor, Maine

Mushrooms, Sausage and Pasta

"Quick, easy and very good!"

Preparation Time: 20 minutes

4 servings

8	ounces hot or sweet Italian sausage
2	cloves garlic
1½	cups sliced mushrooms
1	28-ounce can plum tomatoes
1	teaspoon sugar
¾	teaspoon salt
1	pound favorite pasta

Brown sausage (with casings removed) and 2 minced garlic cloves over medium-high heat. Add mushrooms and cook until browned. Stir in plum tomatoes, sugar and salt. Simmer on low, uncovered, 5 to 8 minutes. Cook pasta, drain and return to pot. Add sauce and toss well.

Charlotte LaCrosse
Rockland, Maine

Noodle Pudding

"This can be used as part of a brunch or as a starch with a meal. In our family, this pudding is a must for all holidays and family gatherings, regardless of the season. It is a great leftover reheated in the microwave."

Preparation Time: 30 minutes

Baking Time: 1 hour

12 or more servings

1   pound extra fine egg noodles
2   cups sugar, divided
6   eggs, separated
1   cup milk (whole or skim)
1   pound light cream cheese, room temperature
1   stick butter, softened
4   teaspoons vanilla
    Corn flakes, crushed

Preheat oven to 350°. Cook noodles according to package directions. Drain and set aside. Mix 1⅓ cups sugar, egg yolks and milk. Combine cream cheese, 7 tablespoons butter and vanilla and add to sugar mixture. Beat egg whites until stiff. Add remaining sugar. Fold into mixture. Pour into 3-quart greased casserole. Sprinkle with crushed corn flakes and dot with remaining butter. Bake 1 hour. Cut into squares and serve hot.

Diane Volk
Portland, Maine

Lemon Rice

"This was one of my sister's favorites when she was a caterer in California. She said the lemon added a lovely aroma as well as a fresh taste. Makes a delicious companion to chicken."

Preparation Time: 10 minutes

Cooking Time: 25 minutes

6 servings

1½ cups uncooked rice
2   tablespoons butter
¼   cup dry vermouth (optional)
2¼ cups chicken broth (increase by ¼ if not using vermouth)
¾   teaspoon salt
     Pinch pepper
     Grated rind of 1 lemon
2   tablespoons fresh minced parsley

Sauté rice in butter. Do not brown. Add vermouth, chicken broth, salt and pepper. Bring to a boil. Stir. Cover tightly and reduce heat to lowest setting. Cook 25 minutes, stirring occasionally. Toss rice with grated lemon peel and fresh parsley. Serve.

Ann Dynan
Greenwich, Connecticut

Beans and Rice

Preparation Time: 15 minutes

4 servings

⅛   pound salt pork (remove rind, cut into tiny pieces)
1   8-ounce can tomato sauce
2   teaspoons adobo seasoning*
2½ teaspoons sofrito*
1   teaspoon garlic powder
1   15½-ounce can red kidney beans
    Cooked rice

Fry salt pork pieces until just brown, 5 minutes. Add tomato sauce, adobo seasoning, and garlic powder. Let simmer. Add beans with juice and sofrito. Heat through. Serve on individual servings of rice.

Erna Johnson
Old Orchard Beach, Maine

Tester's Note: *Both sofrito and adobo seasoning are available in the ethnic section of the supermarket. For a less salty taste, pour boiling water over the salt pork before frying.

Brown Rice, Broccoli and Feta Cheese Bake

"Even for those who are not vegetarians, this is a wonderfully tasty dish."

Preparation Time: 50 minutes

4 servings

1	cup white or brown rice
2	cups water
½	teaspoon salt
2	teaspoons vegetable oil
¼	cup olive oil
4	garlic cloves, minced
2	medium tomatoes, diced
1	bunch broccoli, stalks peeled and cut into bite size pieces, about 5 cups
½	teaspoon oregano
¼	cup water
1	cup olives, halved (optional)
1	cup crumbled feta cheese, about 5 ounces
	Fresh ground pepper

Combine the rice, water, salt and vegetable oil in saucepan and bring to a boil over high heat. Lower heat to simmer and cook until all the water is absorbed, 20 minutes for white rice, 45 minutes for brown. When rice is done, remove from heat and keep covered. In large skillet, heat olive oil over medium heat. Sauté garlic for about 2 minutes, stirring frequently. Do not brown. Add tomatoes and sauté an additional 2 minutes. Add broccoli and oregano. Toss well. Pour in water and add olives. Cover pan. Raise heat to medium high and cook for 5 minutes or until broccoli is tender, but not mushy. Remove cover and toss mixture. Stir in hot rice, feta cheese and black pepper. Serve immediately.

Eleanor Allen
Freedom, Maine

Tester's Note: The olives add quite a lot to this recipe. I would suggest using kalamata olives.

Orzo with Parmesan and Basil

Preparation Time: 10 minutes

Cooking Time: 25 minutes

4 servings

3　tablespoons butter
1½　cups orzo
3　cups chicken broth
½　cup grated Parmesan cheese
1½　teaspoons dried basil, crumpled (or 1 tablespoon chopped
　　fresh basil)
　　Salt and pepper

Melt butter in skillet at medium high heat. Add orzo and sauté until it starts to turn brown. Add stock and bring to boil. Reduce heat, cover and simmer until liquid is absorbed and orzo is tender, about 20 minutes. Mix in cheese and basil. Season with salt and pepper.

Sally Sewall
South Portland, Maine

Tester's Note: Delicious as a side dish.

Risotto with Lobster and Spinach

"A wonderful friend prepared this for my birthday last year. We sat at sunset, looking out at the peaceful lake and enjoyed this taste treat. I loved the dish so much that I have prepared it several times for holidays and special occasions. Thank you, Julia!"

Preparation Time: 50 to 60 minutes

6 servings

1	cup dry white wine
5	cups chicken broth
2	tablespoons butter
2	tablespoons olive oil
1	pound freshly cooked lobster, cut into chunks
8	ounces fresh shiitake mushrooms, stems removed, sliced
1	cup finely-chopped onion
2	cloves garlic, minced
1½	cups Arborio rice, uncooked
8	ounces fresh spinach leaves, tough stems removed
½	cup freshly grated Parmesan cheese
½	teaspoon dried basil
	Fresh ground pepper

Combine wine and chicken broth in a saucepan; bring to a boil. Reduce heat to low, and keep warm. Heat 1 tablespoon butter in fry pan over low heat. Add lobster chunks and warm slowly, turning lobster to coat all sides in butter. When warm, remove from heat and set aside, covered. Melt remaining butter in large saucepan. Add oil and sauté mushrooms, onion and garlic over medium-high heat, stirring constantly, until vegetables are tender. Add rice; stir well. Add 1 cup broth and wine mixture; cook over medium heat, stirring constantly, until most of the liquid is absorbed. Continue adding broth mixture, ½ cup at a time, and cook stirring frequently, until mixture is creamy and rice is tender. (The entire process should take 30 to 35 minutes.) Stir in spinach, lobster, ⅓ cup cheese, and basil. Cover and let stand 2 to 3 minutes. Sprinkle with additional cheese and pepper. Serve immediately.

Kathleen Leslie
Cape Elizabeth, Maine

vegetables, pickles & Relishes

Asparagus Casserole

"A friend, Grace Spingler, of Longmeadow, Massachusetts, gave me this recipe many years ago. It is easy to adjust the recipe to serve two. Great for family dinner, company dinner and pot luck suppers!"

Preparation Time: 15 minutes

Baking Time: 30 minutes

6 servings

3   14½-ounce cans cut asparagus
1   stick butter or margarine, melted
1½ cups crumbs from buttery-style crackers
⅔   cup grated, sharp cheddar cheese
¾   cup chopped pecans

Preheat oven to 350°. Drain asparagus, saving ½ cup juice. Combine melted butter with cracker crumbs. In a greased 1½ to 2-quart casserole dish make layers of asparagus, cheese, then crumbs. Sprinkle top with pecans and spoon the reserved asparagus liquid over top. Bake for 30 minutes.

Suzanne Dolloff
Standish, Maine

Variation: Our tester steamed 1½ pounds of fresh asparagus for 10 minutes and found that it worked well in this easy, elegant dish.

Crockpot Baked Beans

"This was my Mom's recipe - a French one - and every Saturday night we had these with potato salad, hot dogs and hot rolls. My husband had Alzheimer's and passed away on January 2, 1999 and he sure loved these beans! With the help of the Agency on Aging and others, I cared for him in my home for 3 years after we found out he had it."

Preparation Time: 15 minutes

Cooking Time: 6 to 9 hours

5 to 6 servings

2	pounds pea beans
¼	pound salt pork, diced
1	large onion, chopped
½	cup sugar
¾	cup molasses
1	teaspoon salt
2	teaspoons dry mustard
1	tablespoon pepper
2	teaspoons Worcestershire sauce (optional)
½	cup catsup (optional)

Rinse and clean beans. Parboil 2 minutes. Turn burner off and let set 1 hour. Then drain. Bring 2 quarts of water to a boil. Put beans in crock pot and add salt pork and onion. Cover beans with boiling water, molasses and remaining ingredients. Set on high and leave plugged in for 6 to 9 hours. Peek in from time to time and, if using up water too quickly, change setting to low.

Elizabeth P. Beaulieu
Woodland, Maine

Tester's Note: Increasing the amount of molasses by ⅔ cup gives these delicious beans even more color and flavor.

vegetarian chili

"This is a quick and easy meal that is wonderful served with biscuits."

Preparation Time: 15 minutes

Cooking Time: 10 minutes

4 to 6 servings

2   14½-ounce cans herb-flavored tomatoes
1   15½-ounce can kidney beans, drained and rinsed
1   15½-ounce can black beans, drained and rinsed
1   15¼-ounce can whole kernel corn, drained
1   tablespoon chili powder

Mix all ingredients in a saucepan and heat through. Try to prepare a day ahead to let the flavors blend; reheat the next day.

Jill Wyman
Belfast, Maine

Tester's Note: This colorful, tasty dish is also good served cold on top of a bed of lettuce.

Harvard Beets

"My mother always made this at Thanksgiving. I think of her every time I make it."

Preparation Time: 20 minutes

10 servings

2	15-ounce cans sliced beets
2	tablespoons butter
1	tablespoon cornstarch
¼	cup sugar
½	teaspoon salt
⅓	teaspoon vinegar
½	teaspoon minced onions

Drain beets, saving liquid. Melt butter, blend in cornstarch. Add beet liquid and stir constantly over direct heat until sauce boils and thickens. Add remaining ingredients and beets and continue heating slowly until beets are hot enough to serve.

Edwina S. Bonney
Turner, Maine

Note: 5 cups of cooked, sliced fresh beets may be used, substituting water for the beet juice and adding a little red food coloring.

Scalloped Broccoli

"A recipe from a friend that I really liked."

Preparation Time: 20 minutes

Baking Time: 35 to 45 minutes

4 to 6 servings

2   pounds fresh broccoli
4   eggs, beaten
1   cup mayonnaise
2   10¾-ounce cans cream of mushroom soup
2   cups grated cheddar cheese
2   tablespoons onion flakes
     Salt and pepper to taste
1   stick of butter, melted
1   cup crumbled buttery crackers

Preheat oven to 350°. Steam or boil broccoli until just tender. Drain. Combine eggs, mayonnaise, soup, cheese, onion flakes and seasonings and mix in the broccoli. Pour into a greased 2 to 3-quart casserole. Mix butter and cracker crumbs and sprinkle over casserole. Bake, uncovered, for 35 to 45 minutes.

Hilary Clark
Portland, Maine

Sweet and Sour Red Cabbage

"Dad did a good bit of the cooking at our house, and because he loved cabbage, we ate a lot of it. He especially liked it left over, mixed with cut-up potatoes and beef, simmered in gravy in a cast-iron skillet. This he called "kleek" - some adaptation, we always thought, of words from Dutch, his native language. This red cabbage recipe was always served with turkey or duck at Thanksgiving and Christmas."

Preparation Time: 15 to 20 minutes

Baking Time: 1½ hours

6 to 8 servings

1	medium red cabbage, finely shredded
½	cup cold water
½	cup white vinegar
2	tablespoons butter
1	teaspoon salt
3	tablespoons sugar

Preheat oven to 350°. Put cabbage in a greased 3-quart baking dish with a cover. Pour water and vinegar over cabbage. Sprinkle with salt and sugar. Dot with butter. Cover and bake 1½ hours, stirring once or twice.

Kay White
Portland, Maine

Carrot and Pea Casserole

"I thought this recipe had been lost since my mother (who has Alzheimer's disease) no longer remembers. I went through her homemade cookbook and found it! When asked for a recipe, this is the first thing I thought of since I loved it so much as a child. It is graded 'Delicious' in her cookbook and is from her mother (my grandmother). Another reason I want to pass it along to others is that is it an Acadian French dish and was always prepared for our Acadian family at Christmas, Easter and big family gatherings."

Preparation Time: 30 minutes

Baking Time: 1½ hours

6 to 8 servings

¼ cup chopped onions
4 tablespoons butter
4 slices dry or toasted bread, broken into pieces (1½ cups)
  Boiling water
1½ cups cooked, diced carrots
1½ cups cooked peas (fresh, frozen or canned and drained)
1 cup evaporated milk
½ cup vegetable liquids (from canned veggies), or vegetable
  stock
  Salt and pepper to taste
3 eggs, well beaten

Preheat oven to 350°. In saucepan cook onions in butter until soft. Add bread pieces and enough boiling water to moisten the bread well. Add onions, carrots, peas, milk and vegetable liquids (or stock), salt and pepper. Stir in eggs and pour into a greased 1½-quart baking dish. Cover and place in a pan of water in oven for about 1½ hours, or until a knife inserted in middle comes out clean.

Diane Voisine
Fort Kent, Maine

chard and Red Potato Lasagna

"Serve this wonderful dish with grilled meat, chicken or fish. It combines leafy greens with a starch!"

Preparation Time: 30 minutes

Baking Time: 1 hour and 15 minutes

4 to 6 servings

6   medium red potatoes
1   clove garlic
1½ teaspoons salt
    Freshly ground pepper to taste
6½ tablespoons butter
18 chard leaves
2-3 ounces Swiss cheese, shredded
¼   cup cream

Preheat oven to 350°. Slice potatoes as thin as possible. Grease a 3-quart baking dish and rub with garlic. Layer ⅓ of the potatoes in baking dish; sprinkle with ⅓ of the salt and pepper. Dot with 1½ tablespoons butter. Layer ⅓ chard leaves. Sprinkle ⅓ of the cheese over chard. Repeat layers 2 more times, ending with cheese. Dot with remaining butter, pour cream over top, cover and bake for 1 hour and 15 minutes or until potatoes are soft.

Rebecca Hotelling
Freeport, Maine

Delicious— would be fun for a party — Aug. 8, 2012

Corn Scallop

"Here's a very good and quick vegetable casserole, enjoyed for many years in our family. The following is a hint about vegetables from a Home Comfort Cook Book, established in 1864: 'Spinach may be the broom of the stomach, but sauerkraut is the vacuum cleaner.'"

Preparation Time: 30 minutes

Baking Time: 45 to 60 minutes

4 to 6 servings

½ cup chopped onion
½ cup chopped green pepper
1 tablespoon butter
2 eggs, separated
2 tablespoons sugar
   Salt and pepper to taste
1 14¾-ounce can creamed corn
½ cup cracker crumbs

Preheat oven to 350°. Sauté onions and peppers in butter. In a bowl beat egg yolks and add sugar, salt, pepper, onions, green pepper and canned corn. Add cracker crumbs and mix well. Beat egg whites until stiff peaks form. Fold into corn mixture. Pour into greased casserole; set casserole in a pan of water and bake for 45 to 60 minutes, or until knife blade inserted into center comes out clean.

Glenna Leavitt
Howland, Maine

Italian Caponata

Preparation Time: 1 hour

8 servings

2	pounds fresh eggplant, cut into 1-inch cubes
1	tablespoon salt
3	tablespoons olive oil, divided
2	cups coarsely chopped celery
1	cup chopped carrot
¾	cup chopped yellow onion
⅓	cup wine vinegar
4	teaspoons sugar
1	28-ounce can crushed tomatoes
2	tablespoons tomato paste
6	green olives, chopped
2	tablespoons capers
4-5	anchovies, packed in oil but drained, chopped
	Salt and pepper to taste

Dust eggplant with salt and allow to drain in a colander.
Meanwhile, in large frying pan heat 2 tablespoons olive oil.
Sauté celery, carrot and onion about 15 minutes. Place mixture in
heavy 2-quart saucepan. In frying pan, heat remaining tablespoon
olive oil. Add drained eggplant and sauté for 10 minutes. Add
eggplant to saucepan. Add vinegar, sugar, tomatoes, tomato paste,
olives, capers and anchovies. Simmer for 15 to 20 minutes.
Add salt and pepper. Chill and serve.

The Honorable John Baldacci, U.S. Congressman
Bangor, Maine

**Tester's Note: This was excellent served cold with barbequed
chicken breasts. There was enough left to pour over lightly-
sautéed chicken breasts. Bake, uncovered at 325° for 40 minutes,
and serve over pasta. Also delicious! We omitted the anchovies
and still enjoyed this tasty dish.**

Middle-Eastern Style Okra

"This is a quick, nutritious and unusually simple dish based on a recipe from a Syrian friend. It's excellent served with basmati rice and chicken, fish, or lamb."

Preparation Time: 20 minutes

4 servings

2   tablespoons olive oil or butter
½   teaspoon black onion seeds or black mustard seeds
2½   cups whole okra (the smaller the better!), washed
2   cloves garlic, minced
¼   cup water (optional)
1½   cups canned, ground tomatoes
2   teaspoons freshly-squeezed lemon juice
        Salt and pepper to taste

Heat skillet over medium-high heat and add oil or butter. Add black onion or black mustard seeds and cook until the seeds "pop". Turn heat down to medium. Add okra and garlic, cover the pan and cook 3 to 5 minutes. Look in pan after 2 to 3 minutes to make sure the garlic does not burn. If garlic is browning, lower heat, add ¼ cup water, and continue cooking. Add tomatoes and lemon juice. Simmer for 5 minutes, or until okra is soft but not mushy. Season with salt and pepper. Can be served warm or cold.

Mary Taddia
Portland, Maine

Eggplant and Tomato au Gratin

Preparation Time: 20 minutes

4 servings

1	medium eggplant
1-2	tablespoons olive oil
2	large, ripe tomatoes, sliced
	Salt, pepper and fresh herbs (optional)
¼-⅓	cup grated cheddar or Parmesan cheese

Preheat broiler. Slice eggplant and sauté slices on both sides in olive oil. When browned remove slices from pan and drain well on paper towels. Place slices in a broiler-proof pan and place a tomato slice on each eggplant slice. Sprinkle grated cheese on top of tomatoes and run under broiler to melt cheese.

Sheila Donaldson
Falmouth, Maine

Onion Casserole

Preparation Time: 10 minutes

Baking Time: 30 minutes

6 servings

4	cups sliced sweet onion
1	stick margarine or butter, divided
1¼	cups cornbread stuffing mix
1	10¾-ounce can cream of mushroom soup
¼	cup sour cream

Preheat oven to 350°. In saucepan sauté onions in 6 tablespoons butter until limp. Stir in 1 cup stuffing mix, soup and sour cream. Spoon into greased 1½ to 2-quart casserole. Top with remaining stuffing mix and dot with remaining butter. Bake for 30 minutes, or until lightly browned.

Sally Ferko
Erie, Pennsylvania

Creamed Onions

"A must at Thanksgiving."

Preparation Time: 45 minutes

Baking Time: 30 minutes

8 to 10 servings

4	tablespoons butter or oil
4	tablespoons flour
1½-2	cups milk (regular or soy)
1	envelope cream of leek soup mix
2	16-ounce jars small onions
	Parsley, salt and pepper to taste

Preheat oven to 350°. Make a cream sauce by melting butter over low heat and stirring in flour. Stirring constantly, slowly add milk until you get a smooth consistency. Stir in soup mix. Drain onions and add to milk mixture; add seasonings to taste. Put in a greased casserole dish and bake, covered, for 30 minutes, or until bubbly.

Bambi Jones
Alna, Maine

Tester's Note: This easy dish can be cooked a day ahead and reheated.

Potato Melody

Preparation Time: 15 minutes

Baking Time: 1 hour

6 to 8 servings

1   32-ounce bag frozen hash brown potatoes
½   10¾-ounce can cream of mushroom soup
1   cup sour cream
1   cup grated cheddar cheese
¼   cup melted butter or margarine, divided
¼   cup chopped onion
1   cup crushed corn flakes

Preheat oven to 350°. Combine first 4 ingredients. Add
2 tablespoons melted butter/margarine and onion. Pour into
a greased 13x9x2-inch baking dish. Top with corn flakes and
remaining butter/margarine. Bake for 1 hour.

Ann Bonney
Portland, Maine

**Note: This dish may be assembled a day or two in advance and
refrigerated until ready to bake.**

Kugelis (Grated Potato Pudding)

"This recipe has been in our family for many years. It was brought over from Lithuania and was always served on special occasions as a side dish with a topping of sour cream on each slice or square. It can be reheated the next day in a microwave oven or can be warmed in a frying pan. Hope you enjoy it!"

Preparation Time: 45 minutes

Baking Time: 1¼ to 1½ hours

10 to 12 servings

6   slices bacon, diced
1   medium onion, diced
3   eggs
6-8 large white potatoes
1   12-ounce can evaporated milk
2   teaspoons salt
1   teaspoon pepper

Preheat oven to 375 °. Fry bacon until soft. Add onion and continue frying until onion is soft. Set aside to cool. Beat eggs in a separate bowl. Peel, and then grate, potatoes into a large bowl. Pour off some of the starch liquid from the potatoes and pour evaporated milk over them. Stir together bacon and onion mixture, eggs, salt and pepper. Add to potatoes and stir well. Pour into a greased 9x13-inch pan. Bake for 1¼ to 1½ hours or until lightly browned.

Virginia Scheckel
Tinley Park, IL

Tester's Note: For the health-conscious cook, use low-fat evaporated milk and cooking spray. It still tastes wonderful.

Irish Colcannon

"This is great with ham!"

Preparation Time: 30 to 35 minutes

4 servings

1	pound potatoes
3	cups finely-cut cabbage
¼	cup butter
½	cup diced onions
¼	cup milk
	Salt and pepper to taste

Peel potatoes and cut into quarters. Cook, covered, in boiling water for 15 to 20 minutes, or until tender. Drain and mash. Meanwhile, cook cabbage until tender in boiling water. Drain. Melt butter in saucepan. Add onions and fry until soft. Add milk and mashed potatoes. Stir until heated through. Add cabbage and beat into mixture over low heat until mixture turns pale green and fluffy. Season with salt and pepper.

Colleen Gurney
Mexico, Maine

Party Potatoes

"My sister makes this dish and raves about it! So, I recently made a double batch for a family gathering and it was a big hit! I always love a recipe you can make ahead."

Preparation Time: 45 minutes

Baking Time: 30 minutes

6 to 8 servings

8-10	medium all-purpose potatoes
1	8-ounce carton sour cream
1	8-ounce package cream cheese, softened
4	tablespoons butter
1	teaspoon onion salt (or ⅓ cup chopped chives)
	Salt and pepper to taste
	Paprika

Preheat oven to 350°. Peel potatoes. Cut into 1-inch cubes. Boil until very tender (about 25 minutes). Beat sour cream and cream cheese together in large bowl. Add hot potatoes. Beat until smooth. Add butter, onion salt, salt and pepper. Pour into well-greased casserole. Sprinkle with paprika. Bake, covered, for 15 minutes; bake, uncovered, for another 15 minutes or more, if dish has been refrigerated. (Can be made ahead and refrigerated until baking.)

Peggy Thompson
South Portland, Maine

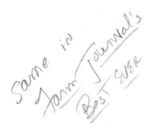

Potato Latkes (Pancakes)

"Potato pancakes are the traditional dish of Chanukah, the Jewish holiday. They supplement the ritual of candle lighting during this time. My dad loved potato latkes and I have demonstrated and made these for many elementary school classes while teaching in the Portland schools."

Preparation Time: 30 minutes

40 3-inch pancakes

6	large Idaho potatoes, peeled
3	medium onions, peeled
4	eggs, lightly beaten
¼-½	cup flour
	Salt to taste
	Freshly ground black pepper
	Canola oil for frying

Grate potatoes, using largest holes on hand grater (or, in food processor, dice first, then process slightly with steel blade). With each potato grate or process half an onion. Place grated vegetables in sieve and press out excess moisture. Discard liquid. Beat eggs into potato-onion mixture. Add enough flour to make light batter. Add salt and pepper. Heat ¼-inch oil in heavy skillet. Drop 2 tablespoons batter into oil and flatten. Fry for 2 minutes, or until crisp; then turn and fry on other side. (For thicker pancakes with soft interior, do not flatten and/or use slightly larger amount.) Remove pancakes with spatula and place on paper towels to drain.

Susan Nielsen
Portland, Maine

Sweet Potato Pancakes

"There is no way to make a potato pancake crispy other than frying it in butter. At least the added sweet potato is extra good for you!"

Preparation Time: 30 minutes

4 to 6 servings

1	cup grated white potato, firmly packed
1	cup grated sweet potato, firmly packed
1	cup grated carrot, firmly packed
2	tablespoons grated onion
¼	cup chopped parsley
4	eggs, beaten
⅓	cup flour
1	teaspoon salt
	Freshly ground black pepper to taste
	Juice of ½ lemon
	Dash of nutmeg
	Optional: 1 small clove garlic, crushed
	Yogurt or sour cream as garnish
	Fresh chives, chopped as garnish

Place grated white potato and sweet potato in a colander over a bowl. Salt lightly and let stand 15 minutes. Rinse and squeeze out well to get rid of all the water. Combine all ingredients and mix well. Fry in butter in a heavy skillet until browned and crisp. Serve immediately, topped with yogurt or sour cream and chives.

Vera Berv
Scarborough, Maine

Baked Sweet Potatoes with Roasted Pecans and Easy Cinnamon-Orange Sauce

"These are simply beautiful (colorful) and beautifully simple. Jewel yams, the ones with purple skin, are my favorites."

Preparation Time: 10 minutes

Baking Time: 30 minutes

4 servings

4　　medium sweet potatoes
¼　　cup pecans, coarsely chopped
　　　Dash of ground cinnamon
¼　　cup orange juice concentrate, thawed

Preheat oven to 400°. Scrub sweet potatoes well, remove any spots and poke each several times with a fork. Bake for 30 minutes, removing when potatoes yield easily to an inserted fork. Meanwhile, roast pecans in a regular or toaster oven for 5 to 10 minutes at 350°, or until fragrant and lightly browned. Slice halfway into each potato with a lengthwise cut, peel back skin a bit and fluff insides with a fork. Sprinkle cinnamon and then 1 tablespoon juice concentrate evenly across each potato. Top with roasted pecans.

Vera Berv
Scarborough, Maine

My Sweet Potato Casserole

"This is a perfect recipe for pot luck dinners."

Preparation Time: 45 minutes

Baking Time: 1 hour

6 servings

4	medium sweet potatoes, boiled, peeled and mashed
4	apples, cored and sliced, not peeled
½	cup dried apricots, sliced
¼	cup grated fresh ginger
	Cinnamon to taste
	Ground cloves to taste

Preheat oven to 350°. In a greased 2 to 3-quart casserole, layer ingredients as follows: sweet potatoes, apples, apricots, sweet potatoes, apples . Sprinkle each layer with ginger, cinnamon and cloves. Sprinkle the final apple layer with cinnamon only. Bake for 1 hour.

Mary Hillas
Falmouth, Maine

Southern Squash

"A Thanksgiving specialty"

Preparation Time: 20 minutes

Baking Time: 1 hour

8 to 10 servings

3	pounds hubbard squash, peeled, seeded and cubed
½	cup chopped onions
	Dash of pepper
1	teaspoon salt
2	eggs, lightly beaten
4	tablespoons butter
1	tablespoon sugar

Preheat oven to 375°. Boil squash until tender; then mash. Add all remaining ingredients. Pour into greased baking dish and bake 1 hour or until golden.

Donna Rubin
Scarborough, Maine

Summer Squash Casserole

"My father and step-mother had a wonderful island vegetable garden every summer in Maine. There was always plenty of squash of all varieties. Boiled new potatoes and this casserole frequently accompanied the lobster picnics they had with family and friends. It was typical to use a mixture of summer squashes, but the dish works equally well using only one variety."

Preparation Time: 30 minutes

Baking Time: 35 to 40 minutes

6 to 8 servings

- 2 pounds summer squash (zucchini, yellow crookneck and scallop)
- 10 tablespoons butter or margarine, divided
- 1 medium onion, quartered and thinly sliced
  Salt and pepper to taste
- 1 cup cubed, fresh white bread
- 4-5 ounces Parmesan cheese, freshly grated

Preheat oven to 350°. Steam squash until partially cooked. Slice about ¼-inch thick. Melt 1 stick butter and sauté onions until soft. Butter 13x9x2-inch baking dish. Add a layer of squash, combining all kinds. Lightly salt and pepper and cover with a layer of buttery onions and Parmesan cheese. Repeat these layers 2 more times. Melt 2 tablespoons butter and mix in bread cubes. Spread bread mixture over the top of the casserole and sprinkle liberally with Parmesan cheese. Bake, uncovered, for 35 to 40 minutes, or until bubbly and lightly browned.

Deborah Dillon
Brunswick, Maine

Note: This dish may be assembled earlier in the day and refrigerated until ready to bake.

zucchiní-Eggplant creole

"Originally from the __Joy of Cooking__, this recipe was changed each time it was passed from neighbor to neighbor. My mother often made this dish for company because everyone liked it. It reminds me of her good, healthy cooking and her love of beauty. The food on the sideboard buffet was always pretty as well as delicious."

Preparation Time: 30 minutes

Baking Time: 30 minutes

6 servings

1   medium eggplant, peeled and diced
     Boiling water
4   tablespoons butter, divided
3.   tablespoons flour
3   large tomatoes, peeled and chopped (or 2 cups canned
        tomatoes)
1   small green pepper, seeded and chopped
1   small onion, peeled and chopped
½   small zucchini, sliced or chopped
½   small yellow summer squash, sliced or chopped
1   teaspoon salt
1   tablespoon brown sugar
½   bay leaf
2   cloves
1   cup bread crumbs

Preheat oven to 350°. Cook eggplant in boiling water for 10 minutes. Drain and place in greased 3-quart baking dish. In sauce pan, over medium heat, melt 3 tablespoons butter. Add onion and sauté for 1 or 2 minutes, stirring. Add flour; cook and stir until blended. Add remaining vegetables, salt, sugar, bay leaf and cloves. Cook 5 minutes, then pour over eggplant. Melt remaining tablespoon butter and stir in bread crumbs. Sprinkle over eggplant mixture. Bake for 30 minutes.

Joan Dinsmore
Portland, Maine

zucchini and corn casserole

"The first time I met my new neighbor, Cecile Grotton, she had just signed up as a RSVP volunteer and had invited another staff member and me for lunch. This recipe is what she had prepared - delicious! I have shared this with many others over the past 20 years."

Preparation Time: 25 minutes

Baking Time: 45 minutes

6 servings

1	onion, chopped
3	cups sliced, unpeeled zucchini
2	tablespoons butter, divided
3	eggs, beaten
1	15¼-ounce can whole kernel corn
8	ounces grated sharp cheddar cheese
8	ounces grated mozzarella cheese
	Salt and pepper to taste
1	tablespoon butter
½-¾	cup bread crumbs

Preheat oven to 350°. In saucepan melt 1 tablespoon butter and sauté onion and zucchini until softened. Cool. Mix in next 4 ingredients and place mixture in a greased 2-quart casserole. Melt remaining butter, stir in bread crumbs and sprinkle over zucchini mixture. Bake for 45 minutes.

Thelma C. Andrews
Brewer, Maine

Tester's Note: If you cook zucchini and onions until slightly browned, it gives this tasty casserole a beautiful golden color.

Baked Plum Tomatoes

"Try these tomatoes as a party dish. They can be cooking before, or as, your guests arrive and served warm or at room temperature."

Preparation Time: 5 minutes

Baking Time: 45 to 60 minutes

4 servings

6	fresh plum tomatoes
¼	cup fine bread crumbs
2	tablespoons chopped fresh oregano
	Salt and pepper to taste
2	tablespoons olive oil

Preheat oven to 350°. Wash and dry tomatoes. Cut in half lengthwise. In small bowl mix crumbs, oregano, salt and pepper. Coat 11x7x1½-inch baking dish with olive oil. Add the tomatoes, sliding them about to completely coat them with oil. Arrange them cut side up and sprinkle each half with crumb mixture. Bake 45 to 60 minutes.

Janet Richardson
Portland, Maine

Grilled Tomatoes with Pesto

Preparation Time: 15 minutes

6 servings

3   medium to firm tomatoes, cored and halved crosswise
¼   cup pesto
6   very thin onion slices
½   cup shredded Monterey Jack cheese (about 2 ounces)
⅓   cup smoked almonds, chopped
2   tablespoons minced parsley

Preheat grill to medium. Using a spoon, hollow out the top ¼-inch of tomato halves. Top each tomato half with 2 teaspoons pesto and an onion slice. Arrange tomatoes in 2 foil pans. Place on grill, cover and grill for 8 to 10 minutes, or until tomatoes are heated through. In mixing bowl, stir together cheese, almonds and parsley. Sprinkle over tomatoes. Cover and grill about 5 minutes more, or until cheese melts.

Sally Sewall
South Portland, Maine

Tangy Oven-Roasted Vegetables

Preparation Time: 25 to 30 minutes

Baking Time: 45 minutes

6 to 8 servings

2	potatoes, cut into 1-inch chunks
2	sweet potatoes, peeled and cut into 1-inch chunks
2	carrots, peeled and cut into 1-inch chunks
1	large onion, cut into wedges
1	medium zucchini, cut into 1-inch chunks
2	bell peppers (1 red, 1 green), cut into 1-inch squares
⅓	cup low-sodium soy sauce
⅓	cup rice wine vinegar
1	tablespoon grated fresh ginger root
1	tablespoon honey
1	tablespoon dark sesame oil
3	garlic cloves, minced
½	teaspoon ground anise, or crushed anise seeds (optional)

Preheat oven to 425°. Parboil potatoes, sweet potatoes and carrots in boiling water to cover for 2 minutes. Drain. In large bowl, combine with onions, zucchini and peppers. Whisk remaining ingredients together. Pour over vegetables and toss well. Place vegetables in single layer on large lightly-oiled baking tray or broiler pan. Bake, stirring frequently, until all vegetables are tender, about 45 minutes.

Kathleen Leslie
Cape Elizabeth, Maine

Note: Many vegetable combinations are possible in this healthy, colorful dish. Have fun experimenting!

veggie casserole

Preparation Time: 45 to 60 minutes

Baking Time: 35 to 40 minutes

8 servings

1½ cups coarsely chopped cauliflower, cooked and drained
1½ cups peas, fresh or frozen, cooked and drained
1½ cups coarsely chopped broccoli, cooked and drained
1   cup chunked carrots, cooked and drained
½   cup coarsely chopped onions
1   cup chopped celery
½   cup water chestnuts, halved or sliced
1   10¾-ounce can condensed celery soup
1   cup grated cheddar cheese
1   cup sour cream
    Salt and pepper to taste
½   cup bread crumbs
2   tablespoons butter or margarine, melted

Preheat oven to 350°. Place vegetables, in order given in greased 2-quart casserole. In small bowl, combine soup, cheese and sour cream. Blend and season with salt and pepper. Pour over veggies. Combine bread crumbs and melted butter/margarine. Sprinkle over top. Cover and bake 20 minutes. Uncover and bake 15 to 20 minutes longer.

Linda Johnson
Eastport, Maine

Tester's Note: This dish is wonderful served with rice, which blends with any extra "juices" from the veggies.

Zucchini Relish

"I make this every year. We love it with everything."

Preparation Time: 30 minutes

Cooking Time: 30 minutes

6 to 8 pints

12	cups shredded zucchini
2	green peppers, seeded and sliced thin
2	red peppers, seeded and sliced thin
4	cups thinly-sliced onions
5	tablespoons canning salt
2½	cups vinegar
¾	tablespoon corn starch
6	cups sugar
½	teaspoon celery seed
¾	teaspoon nutmeg
¾	teaspoon turmeric
½	teaspoon black pepper
1	tablespoon dry mustard

Combine first 5 ingredients and let stand overnight. Next day rinse and drain well. In separate kettle, cook the remaining ingredients to boiling. Add the vegetables to the hot liquid and cook 30 minutes. Seal in hot sterile jars.

Marilyn Tenney
Roque Bluffs, Maine

Dill Pickles

"These are old-fashioned dill pickles, enjoyed for years by the Welch family."

Preparation Time: 45 minutes

6 to 8 quarts

8   pounds cucumbers
8   teaspoons mustard seed
4   teaspoons alum
5   tablespoons dill seeds or bunch of fresh dill
2   quarts water
1   quart vinegar
1   cup canning salt

Wash cucumbers and cut in half lengthwise. Place in each of 6 to 8 hot, sterile quart jars the following: 1 teaspoon mustard seed, ½ teaspoon alum and 2 teaspoons dill seeds or a few sprigs of fresh dill. Bring to a boil the remaining ingredients. Pack cucumbers into the jars. Fill jars to within ½-inch of the top with hot pickling liquid and seal.

Joy and Crystal Welch
Wilton, Maine

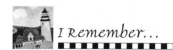

Sweet Pickles

Preparation Time: 45 minutes

Scant 3 quarts

1   46-ounce jar dill pickles
3   cups sugar
½   cup white vinegar
¼   cup pickling spices (tied in small cheesecloth pouch)

Drain pickles, reserving liquid. Cut into slices or chunks. Return to empty pickle jar along with spice pouch. Mix sugar and vinegar and pour over pickles in jar. Add enough reserved dill pickle juice to fill jar. Cover jar and place on counter. Shake daily, turning jar over, for 10 days. Then refrigerate and enjoy.

Catherine B. Houts
Seminole, Florida

Tester's Note: Interesting and pleasant change. Cross between a dill and a sweet pickle. Be sure to wait the 10 days before tasting to get the full flavor.

Our Mother's Green Tomato Pickles

Preparation Time: 30 minutes

Cooking Time: 30 minutes

6 quarts, approximately

1   peck green tomatoes, sliced
3   pounds onions, sliced
½   cup salt
6   cups sugar
3   cups vinegar
1   cup water
¼   cup pickling spice

Sprinkle tomatoes and onions with salt. Let sit overnight.
In morning, drain liquid, add remaining ingredients and cook slowly for 30 minutes. Seal in jars while hot.

Phyllis Scribner and Alan King

Desserts

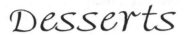

Puddings, Desserts,
Pies, Cakes, Bars,
Cookies & Candy

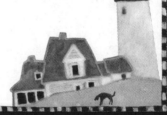

Apple à la Mode

"This recipe is easy and was well-received by my mother's friends when she served it at lunch."

Preparation Time: about 20 minutes

Cooking Time: 4 to 6 minutes

6 servings

1   apple per person
     A touch of butter, about 2 teaspoons
1   tablespoon white or brown sugar

Peel apples and cut into thick wedges. Sauté in a touch of butter, 4 minutes. Flip and sprinkle with sugar to caramelize them. Splash 1 teaspoon water into pan to stop the process. Scoop onto plates and put a little ice cream on top. (Apples are hot when served).

Joan Dinsmore
Portland, Maine

Tester's Note: This simple and delicious recipe could be used for breakfast, without the ice cream, or dessert anytime. Caramelized apples are beautiful to look at as well as eat. I threw in pear slices, which worked well.

Banana Split Cake

Preparation Time: 30 minutes

9 x 13-inch pan

2	cups graham cracker crumbs
1	stick butter
2	cups confectioners' sugar
2	eggs
2	sticks softened margarine
1	teaspoon vanilla
2	cups well drained crushed pineapple
4	large bananas
1	13½-ounce container whipped cream
	Chopped nuts
1	jar Maraschino cherries

Melt butter and mix well with graham cracker crumbs. Press into 9x13-inch pan. Do not bake. Beat together confectioners' sugar, margarine, eggs and vanilla. Beat 20 minutes. Do not under beat. Spread over crumb base. Spread 2 cups well-drained crushed pineapple. Slice 4 or more bananas in thirds lengthwise and layer over pineapple. Spread with whipped topping. Sprinkle with chopped nuts. Decorate with cherries and refrigerate.

Raejean Murphy
Mexico, Maine

Blueberry Buckle

"This was my mother's recipe, a favorite for the whole family. She always made it for family get-togethers after we had gone blueberrying."

Preparation Time: 20 minutes

Baking Time: 45 to 50 minutes

9 x 13-inch pan

¾   cup sugar
¼   cup shortening or margarine
1   egg
½   cup milk
2   cups flour
2   teaspoons baking powder
½   teaspoon salt
2   cups blueberries

Crumb mixture
½   cup sugar
⅓   cup sifted flour
½   teaspoon cinnamon
¼   cup soft butter or margarine

Preheat oven to 375°. Mix thoroughly sugar, shortening and egg (beaten). Stir in milk. Sift together flour, baking powder and salt. Add to the first mixture. Fold in blueberries. Spread batter in greased and floured 9 x 13-inch pan. For Crumb mixture: Combine sugar, flour, cinnamon and butter. Mix until crumbly. Top batter with crumb mixture and bake 45 to 50 minutes. Serve with frozen whipped topping or whipped cream.

Elinor Vigue
Dexter, Maine

Rhubarb Torte

"I always use a glass pan and make sure the egg whites seal the edges. I got this from Inna Anderson in Wisconsin about 1971 and everyone who likes rhubarb loves it. You can get more servings than a pie for your 4 cups of rhubarb."

Preparation Time: 25 minutes or less

Baking Time: 45 minutes

8 to 12 servings

Crust
1¾ cups flour
2 egg yolks
2 tablespoons white sugar
½ cup chopped walnuts
1 teaspoon baking powder
½ cup plus 2 tablespoons shortening

Filling
4 cups rhubarb, cut in ½-inch pieces or smaller
2 egg yolks
1½-1¾ cups white sugar
5 tablespoons flour

Topping
4 egg whites
¾ cup white sugar

Preheat oven to 350° (325° for glass pan). You can use the same mixing bowl for the crust and filling. Mix crust ingredients together with pastry blender. Press into bottom of 9 x 13-inch pan. Combine filling ingredients and spread over crust. Beat 4 egg whites. Add sugar gradually and beat well. Spread over rhubarb filling. Bake 45 minutes.

Sue Winters
South Thomaston, Maine

Tester's Note: This is an unusual rhubarb recipe. It is nice to have another way to prepare it.

chocolate Eclair cake

"This is one of my son Sam's favorite desserts. We make this dessert only for special occasions or when asked to bring it to a family gathering so that it remains a special treat."

Preparation Time: 20 minutes. Make a day ahead.

9 to 12 large servings

Cake
Butter, or nonstick spray
1   box graham crackers
2   3⅛-ounce packages vanilla instant pudding
3   cups milk
1   large container frozen whipped topping, thawed

Frosting
2   ounces unsweetened chocolate (or 6 tablespoons cocoa and
        2 tablespoons vegetable oil)
3   tablespoons butter, melted
2   tablespoons light corn syrup
1   teaspoon vanilla
1½ cups confectioners' sugar
3   tablespoons milk

Butter 9 x 13-inch dish. Layer ⅓ graham crackers on bottom.
In separate bowl, combine puddings and milk. Beat together.
Fold in thawed whipped topping. Pour ½ of this mixture over the layer of crackers. Add second layer of graham crackers and pour remaining mixture over that. Add third layer of graham crackers.
For Frosting: Melt unsweetened chocolate (or mix cocoa with vegetable oil). Add melted butter, corn syrup, vanilla, confectioners' sugar and milk. Stir with spoon. Put frosting on top, then cover and refrigerate overnight.

Sally Subilia
Wells, Maine

cranberry crunch

Preparation Time: 10 to 15 minutes

Baking Time: 45 minutes

4 to 5 servings

1   cup uncooked rolled oats
½   cup flour
¾-1 cup brown sugar
½   cup butter or margarine
1   can whole cranberry sauce

Preheat oven to 350°. Mix together oats, flour and brown sugar. Cut in butter until crumbly. Place ½ of mixture in 8 x 8-inch greased pan. Cover with whole cranberry sauce. Spread rest of crumb mixture evenly on top and bake for 45 minutes. Cut in squares.

Lesa Borg
Biddeford, Maine

Fruit Cobbler in a Skillet

"While stationed at Clovis Air Force Base in Clovis, New Mexico, I acquired this recipe from a good ol' Texas 'gal' who always used fresh peaches or cherries."

Preparation Time: 15 minutes

Baking Time: 40 to 50 minutes

8 servings

1	stick of butter
1	cup sugar
1	cup flour
1	teaspoon baking powder
⅔	cup milk
3	cups fresh fruit, or 1 can of fruit

Preheat oven to 350°. Melt butter in black iron skillet. Mix flour, sugar, and baking powder with milk in bowl. Add melted butter and mix well. Pour back into skillet. To 3 cups of fruit, add sugar to taste, or use a can of fruit. Using all the fruit and juice, pour into the middle of the "batter" in the skillet and bake for 40 to 50 minutes. Serve warm with whipped cream. I like to use a can of peaches when making this.

Elizabeth Douglass
Howland, Maine

Tester's Note: Fresh apples and dried cranberries worked well in this recipe. It must be served from the skillet and not removed whole.

Sugared Fruit cocktail Bake

"My mother would make this recipe whenever she needed a quick dessert for supper. She has been battling with Alzheimer's disease for 10 years."

Preparation Time: 15 minutes

Baking Time: 40 to 45 minutes

10 to 12 servings

1   cup sifted flour
1   cup white sugar
1   teaspoon baking soda
     Dash of salt
1   15¾-ounce can fruit cocktail with juice
1   beaten egg
½   cup brown sugar
½   cup walnuts

Preheat oven to 350°. Mix together flour, white sugar, baking soda and salt. Add fruit cocktail and beaten egg. Pour into greased 9 x 13-inch cake pan. Top with brown sugar and walnuts. Bake for 40 to 45 minutes.

Bella Blier
Frenchville, Maine

Lazy Eclairs

"My future mother-in-law gave me this recipe and it's delicious! I suggest a Pyrex or glass pan for best results. Don't worry if crust seems excessively puffy during cooking. Chocolate, vanilla, butterscotch or even pistachio pudding tastes delicious. For a lighter recipe, substitute sugar or fat-free pudding and Cool Whip. Enjoy!"

Preparation Time: 20 minutes

Baking Time: 30 to 40 minutes

9 x 13-inch pan

Shell/ Crust
1   cup water
1   cup flour
1   stick margarine
4   medium sized eggs

Filling
3   cups milk
2   3½-ounce packages of instant pudding (any flavor)
8   ounces softened cream cheese
1-2 containers whipped topping
     Chocolate syrup

Preheat oven to 375°. In medium saucepan, boil water and margarine. Remove from heat. Add flour. Stir quickly until ball forms. Add eggs one at a time and beat well after each addition. Spread mixture into a 9 x 13-inch greased pan. Bake 30 to 40 minutes until light brown and puffy. Cool. For filling, blend milk with cheese in blender. Mix in pudding. Stir until thick. Pour onto crust. Top with whipped topping, then drizzle with chocolate syrup. Chill for at least 2 hours.

Marla Jandreau
Fort Kent, Maine

Sinful Chocolate Delight

"This recipe was given to me by my grandmother, Tina Bryant from Farmington, New Hampshire."

Preparation Time: 1 hour and 15 minutes

12 servings

1   chocolate cake mix
1½ cups coffee-flavored liqueur or chocolate syrup
2   3⅛-ounce packages of instant chocolate pudding
3   cups milk
     Large container of whipped topping
     Crushed chocolate-covered toffee candy bars

Bake the chocolate cake according to box instructions. Cool cake and break into small squares. Make pudding according to package directions, using only 1½ cups milk per package. Layer ½ of cake squares in bowl. Spread ½ of chocolate syrup or coffee-flavored liqueur on top, then ½ of chocolate pudding. Reserve some toffee candy for top. Spread ½ remaining candy on pudding and top with ½ whipped topping. Repeat layers in above order. Sprinkle reserved candy on top. Refrigerate for at least 2 hours and serve.

Melissa Canwell
Levant, Maine

Wild Maine Blueberry Cobbler

"This recipe is a favorite of all Stonewall Kitchen's out of state guests...It is a way for them to have great wild Maine blueberries, even if they do not live in Maine."

Preparation Time: 30 to 40 minutes

Baking Time: 25 to 30 minutes

6 servings

Butter to grease pan
2	pints rinsed and picked over blueberries or mixed berries OR
2	14-ounce bags frozen blueberries, not defrosted Grated zest of 1 lemon
1	13-ounce jar Stonewall Kitchen Wild Maine Blueberry Jam
½	teaspoon cinnamon
2	cups unbleached all-purpose flour
3	tablespoons sugar
1	tablespoon baking powder
½	teaspoon salt
1	stick unsalted butter, chilled and cut into pieces
½	cup half-and-half or light cream

Preheat oven to 425°. Butter a 2- to 3-quart heavy baking dish. Gently stir blueberries, lemon zest, jam and cinnamon together in a bowl, then pour into prepared dish. Combine flour, 1 tablespoon of sugar, baking powder and salt in food processor and process briefly to blend. Add butter and pulse until mixture resembles coarse meal. Pour in half-and-half and pulse just until dough begins to pull together. Remove dough from processor and knead briefly to form a ball, adding more flour if dough is sticky. Break pieces of dough from ball and cover berries with slightly flattened pieces of dough in a "cobbled" irregular pattern. Sprinkle on remaining sugar. Bake until crust is lightly browned and berries are hot. Remove from oven and let stand for at least 15 minutes before serving. Serve with sweetened whipped cream, vanilla ice cream or yogurt.

Stonewall Kitchen
Portland, Maine

Steamed Cranberry Dessert

"I got this recipe in Minnesota while visiting my brother for Thanksgiving. I made the loaves, wrapped them in foil with a bow and gave them with a nice container of sauce for Christmas gifts with the recipe. A big hit!"

Preparation Time: 10 minutes

Baking Time: 1 hour

4 cakes

3   cups flour
2   cups fresh cranberries
1   cup molasses
4   teaspoons baking soda
1   cup warm water

Sauce
2   cups sugar
1   cup butter
1   cup cream
1   teaspoon vanilla

Preheat oven to 350°. Put flour and cranberries in a bowl. Put molasses in 2-cup measure. Add baking soda and fill to 2 cups with warm water. Pour over flour mixture and stir. Pour into 4 (#2) cans or 4 mini-loaf well-greased pans. Place in pan filled with water to 1-inch from top and cover with foil to steam. Bake for 1 hour. For Sauce: Dissolve sugar in liquids over low heat. Serve warm with sauce on top.

Rev. Judith H. Blanchard
Freeport, Maine

Blackberry Steamed Pudding

"This pudding has been used by three generations in my family and it always brought a smile to my dear husband's face when I served it to him."

Preparation Time: 20 minutes

Steaming Time: 2 hours

6 servings

1	egg
3	tablespoons butter
⅔	cup sugar
1	cup milk
2¼	cups flour
4	teaspoons baking powder
	Salt
1	cup fresh blackberries

Sauce

2	cups water
1½	tablespoons flour
1	cup sugar
1	tablespoon butter
1	teaspoon vanilla

Preheat oven to 350°. Cream butter, sugar and egg. Beat well. Add flour and baking powder alternately with milk and carefully stir in blackberries. Turn into buttered pudding mold or coffee can and steam 2 hours or until done.

For Sauce: Mix sugar and flour in saucepan. Add water and butter. Bring to boil and stir until thick. Add vanilla. Serve hot over pudding. Blackberries can also be put in sauce while cooking.

Genevieve Palmer
Norway, Maine

Tester's Note: I used a deep dish porcelain baking dish set inside a larger dish filled with water and put in a 350° oven. I covered all with a domed lid to catch the steam. It took only 1½ hours to steam and cook since it was flatter than a coffee can.

Bread Pudding

*"Throughout his life my father, Joe, loved desserts.
He always contended that there was a 'separate section' in
the stomach just for desserts and it didn't matter how much
was consumed during the main meal there was always room for
something sweet. He also loved McDonald's milkshakes and in
the last few years of his life we had to take a ride every day to
get one for him."*

Preparation Time: 15 minutes

Baking Time: 1 hour

8 to 10 servings

½   loaf cinnamon / raisin bread
1   apple, cut-up
½   cup baking raisins
3   cups milk
1   package butterscotch pudding (not instant)

Preheat oven to 350°. Cut bread in small cubes, and add apple
and raisins. Pour in 1 cup of milk, mix and let set for 10 minutes.
Mix remaining milk with butterscotch pudding. Pour over bread
mixture. Stir well and bake 1 hour.

Joe Groff
Cape Elizabeth, Maine

Tester's Note: Serve with whipped cream or ice cream.

Butterscotch Bread Pudding

"My mother-in-law gave me this recipe. I had been hunting for one that I really enjoyed for quite some time. This is the best ever! I serve it with frozen whipped topping while still warm."

Preparation Time: 15 to 20 minutes

Baking Time: 45 minutes

6 moderate servings

3	tablespoons butter
½	cup brown sugar
¼	teaspoon baking soda
2	cups milk
2	eggs
	Pinch of salt
2	cups bread cubes

Preheat oven to 350°. Melt butter in medium saucepan, add sugar. Heat until well blended. Dissolve baking soda in milk and add to sugar mixture. Stir until blended. Set aside to cool. Beat eggs lightly, add salt and cooled milk to sugar mixture. Put bread cubes in greased casserole dish and pour the custard mixture over them. Bake for 45 minutes.

Hazel Jollotta
Eastport, Maine

Tester's Note: This "comfort food" would be especially good on a winter night. An interesting addition might include butterscotch chips or raisins.

Honey Orange Bread Pudding

"This is a diabetic recipe and delicious. There are 165 calories in a 4-ounce serving. The exchanges: 1½ starch and 1 fat."

Preparation Time: 10 minutes

Baking Time: 35 to 45 minutes

6 servings

4	slices high fiber bread cut in cubes
6	tablespoons raisins
½	teaspoon cinnamon
3	eggs
¼	cup honey
1½	cups orange juice
1	teaspoon vanilla
¼	teaspoon salt

Preheat oven to 350°. Spray a loaf pan with cooking spray. Combine bread with raisins in loaf pan. Sprinkle with cinnamon and mix well. Combine remaining ingredients in blender or food processor and beat until blended. Pour over bread. Set loaf pan in a larger pan, add boiling water to larger pan. Slide into oven. Bake 35 to 45 minutes or until knife inserted in center comes out clean.

Lorraine Soucy
Saco, Maine

Rice Pudding

"My mother made a rice pudding which I remembered and always loved. I tried for years different recipes but never could duplicate the flavor or texture. About 15 years ago, I found this one. My family just loves it."

Preparation Time: 5 minutes

Baking Time: 2½ hours

4 to 6 servings

¼   cup washed, raw rice, (not instant)
½   cup sugar
¼   teaspoon salt
¼   teaspoon nutmeg
1   teaspoon vanilla
4   cups milk
2   tablespoons butter or margarine
½   cup raisins, (optional) added 1½ hours before pudding
     is done

Preheat oven to 325°. Wash rice well, running it under cold water. Place rice in buttered casserole and add sugar, salt, nutmeg and vanilla. Add cold milk and stir. Add butter or margarine. Bake uncovered for 2½ hours or until rice is tender. Stir occasionally as it cooks. It will become creamy as it cools. Serve with or without cream.

Dorothy Larkin
Cumberland Foreside, Maine

chocolate Mousse

"This is a very simple, quick and delicious recipe."

Preparation Time: 10 minutes

6 servings

1   8-ounce container heavy cream
4   tablespoons sifted Hershey's cocoa
1   jar hot fudge mix (room temperature)

Whip cream. Blend in sifted cocoa and hot fudge mix with wooden spoon. Ready to serve. You can sprinkle chocolate slivers over top for decoration.

Erma Johnson
Old Orchard Beach, Maine

Tester's Note: This is a very smooth, rich mousse and a chocolate lover's delight!

Floating Island

"My children remember visiting their stylish, fun-loving grandmother and enjoying this spectacular dessert with its evocative name. I have adapted her recipe, with the help of Julia Child, to make it easy to prepare in advance and assemble just before serving. Our family now enjoys it for holiday meals, always remembering the special person who introduced us to this delicious, but easy dessert."

Preparation Time: 1 hour and 15 minutes, approximately

Baking Time: 30 to 35 minutes

8 to 10 servings

Meringue
8   egg whites
1   cup sugar
     Pinch salt
¼   rounded teaspoon cream of tartar
¾   teaspoon vanilla

Custard
8   egg yolks
¾   cup sugar
4   cups scalded milk
2   teaspoons vanilla
2   tablespoons Amaretto, Cognac, or other liqueur(optional)

Caramel
1   cup sugar
⅓   cup water

For Meringue: Preheat oven to 250°. Prepare a 3-quart, 3-inch deep baking dish, by buttering and dusting with confectioners' sugar. Using electric mixer, whip 8 egg whites until foamy. Beat in salt and cream of tartar; continue to beat until soft peaks are formed. Beat in 1 cup of sugar, a little at a time, and continue beating until stiff. Beat in vanilla and pour into prepared baking dish. Set in lower middle of oven and bake approximately 30 to

35 minutes, or until toothpick can be inserted and come out clean. Cool on rack. (Can be covered tightly and refrigerated for several days.) For Custard: In 2-quart top of double boiler, using an electric mixer, whisk 8 egg yolks, adding sugar a little at a time. Continue beating until mixture is pale yellow and thick. Add hot milk a little at a time, stirring slowly, but constantly. Set over (not in) hot water. Stir constantly until it thickens to a creamy texture. (Do not overcook and scramble the eggs!) Cool slightly and stir in vanilla and liqueur. (May be refrigerated in covered container for several days).For Caramel: Blend sugar and water in a heavy 6-cup saucepan. (Have large, low pan of cold water nearby in which to quickly cool saucepan of caramel). Bring sugar water to a simmer. Remove from heat and swirl pan by handle until liquid is clear. Return pan to moderately high heat, cover tightly and boil for several minutes, looking occasionally to see if bubbles have become very thick. Uncover and continue boiling and swirling pan slowly until syrup begins to color. Continue until it turns a light caramel color. Remove from heat and continue swirling until mixture darkens to a medium caramel color. Set bottom of pan in cold water to stop cooking. Cool. Caramel will be very hard. (I keep the caramel, stored in the same covered pan, ready to reheat just before serving.) When ready to serve, reheat caramel until it is liquid again. To Serve: Pour custard into a low, rimmed bowl. Loosen meringue and cut into large, irregular pieces for "islands". Arrange on top of the custard sauce. With fork, dribble thin strands of reheated caramel over "islands".

Kathleen Leslie
Cape Elizabeth, Maine

Crème de Caramel

Preparation Time: 30 minutes

Baking Time: 1 hour 45 minutes

8 servings

1   quart heavy cream
1   split vanilla bean
7   egg yolks
2   cups sugar, divided
2   cups water
2   whole eggs

Preheat oven to 250°. Combine the split vanilla bean with heavy cream. Place over high heat and scald the cream. Let cool to room temperature. Place 1 cup sugar with water over high heat and boil until golden brown. Take the caramel from heat and cover the bottoms of eight ramekins. Strain the heavy cream through a sieve to remove the vanilla bean. Take egg yolks and 2 eggs and whisk in 1 cup sugar. Slowly whisk in heavy cream. Ladle cream mixture into ramekins. Place ramekins in a baking pan and add water until it goes half-way up sides of ramekins. Cover with foil and bake. Remove, let cool and serve.

Casa Napoli Ristorante, Daniel Call, Executive Chef
Falmouth, Maine

Note: This recipe is delicious and is really quite easy although it does require constant attention. Keep an eye on the cream. It could get messy if it's not off the heat at the right moment. The same with the caramel, if you miss the golden brown, it will burn in a blink of an eye.

Grapenut Pudding

"Old fashioned puddings are a favorite. I add ½ teaspoon cinnamon and ½ cup raisins to this recipe."

Preparation Time: 10 minutes

Baking Time: 45 minutes

6 to 8 servings

1	quart milk
1	cup grapenuts
3	eggs, beaten
¾	cup sugar
1	teaspoon vanilla
	Pinch of salt

Preheat oven to 350°. Mix milk and grapenuts and let stand. Beat eggs, sugar, vanilla and salt. Add to milk mixture and stir well. Bake 45 minutes.

The Honorable Tom Allen, U.S. Congressman
Portland, Maine

Grace's Cup Custards

"When I was a young child and any of my cousins and I were ill, my Grandmother Grace would always make us what she called cup custards. She reasoned that they were filled with nutritious things and were just sweet enough to seem like a treat. My mother, also Grace, did the same for my children. Recently when my mother, a resident of Sedgewood Commons, was having difficulty eating because of dental problems, and was losing weight at an alarmingly fast rate, I remembered the cup custards. It took me a couple of tries to get them right, but I finally did. She loved them, ate them, gained weight and was strong enough to have the dental problems corrected."

Preparation Time: 10 minutes

Baking Time: 45 minutes to 1 hour

8 to 9 small custard cups

6   eggs
1   quart whole milk
½   cup sugar
1-2 tablespoons vanilla (according to taste)
    Nutmeg

Preheat oven to 370°. Beat eggs on low, add milk, sugar and vanilla. Continue to beat on low until well mixed. Fill each custard cup close to the top with the mixture and sprinkle nutmeg on the top of each custard. Put custard cups in a shallow pan(s) half filled with hot water. Water should come up to within ½-inch of custard cup. Bake in oven for approximately one hour. Because oven temperatures vary, I watch the custard after 45 minutes. To test doneness, insert the handle of a teaspoon or a knife blade into the center. If it comes out clean, custard is done. If you cook the custard too long, it will look like whey. Custards may be served warm or cold, and will keep well in the refrigerator for 5 or 6 days.

Donna Brunstad
Portland, Maine

pudím de coco (coconut custard)

"I received this recipe from Brazilian Jo Hoffman when I was a missionary with the United Church Board for World Ministries in 1973 to '74. It's quick, easy and elegant!"

Preparation Time: 10 minutes

Baking Time: 45 minutes

10 to 12 servings

4   tablespoons sugar
1   14-ounce can sweetened condensed milk
1¾ cups milk
4   eggs
1   cup coconut

Preheat oven to 300°. Blend all ingredients except sugar in a blender or food processor. Put 4 tablespoons sugar in a medium (6 to 8 cup) Corningware dish. Heat, over low heat, stirring until caramelized (be careful not to burn it). Spread around bottom and sides of dish with a spoon. Put contents of blender in pan and bake for about 45 minutes or until solid and a little brown on top. Cool and invert on a dish. Top will be lovely brown caramel.

The Rev. Judith H. Blanchard
Freeport, Maine

Tester's Note: It is not necessary to bake this in a hot water bath, or dip it in hot water to unmold. It can be made, unmolded and refrigerated 24 hours ahead of serving.

Fudge Pudding

"My mother was given this recipe from a friend she taught school with in 1935! It is a yummy dessert."

Preparation Time: about 30 minutes

Baking Time: 20 to 25 minutes

4 to 6 servings

1   cup sugar
½   cup milk
1½ squares unsweetened chocolate
1   tablespoon butter
1   cup bread, small pieces packed down
1   beaten egg
     Nonstick spray

Preheat oven to 350°. Combine sugar, milk, chocolate, and butter in small saucepan and cook until chocolate is melted. Combine bread pieces and egg in large bowl, then add chocolate mixture. Spray an 8 x 8-inch pan. Pour in mixture and bake for 20 to 25 minutes. Serve with whipped cream or hard sauce.

Betsy Hillman
Yarmouth, Maine

Tester's Note: Using 2 squares of chocolate enhanced this recipe.

Pots de crème au chocolat

"As this takes no more than 10 minutes to prepare and serve, and it can be prepared in advance, this sort of "cheat" cuisine (as I call it) tastes far better than similar recipes with an endless list of ingredients and a need for hours of one's time in the kitchen, and allows me to impress guests with my culinary skills and yet not miss a minute of their company."

Preparation Time: 10 minutes

4 to 6 servings

6	ounces semisweet chocolate chips, or plain chocolate broken in small pieces
½	pint light cream
1	egg
	Pinch salt
½	teaspoon vanilla
	Generous dash of orange liqueur, or dark rum (optional)

Put chocolate in food processor. Heat cream until just under boiling point, then pour over the chocolate. Blend until smooth (the heat of the cream will melt the chocolate). Add the egg, salt, vanilla essence, and liqueur or rum (if desired) and blend again quickly. Pour the thin mixture into small pots or glasses and chill in the 'fridge several hours or overnight when mixture will be firm. Serve plain or garnish with grated chocolate or mint leaf.

Melody MacDonald
Scarborough, Maine

Note: This dessert is equally wonderful using liquid egg substitute.

Poor Man's Pudding

"This recipe can be mixed and cooked in the same oven-proof bowl. It's very simple and delicious. It tastes the same as the French "Beignets" or dumplings in syrup with much less fuss. This recipe goes back 4 to 5 generations if not more. It is a French Acadian recipe."

Preparation Time: 10 to 15 minutes

Baking Time: 30 minutes

6 to 8 servings

Syrup
1½ cups water
1   cup brown sugar
⅓   cup butter

Batter
½   cup sugar
1   cup flour
⅓   teaspoon salt
2   teaspoons baking powder
½   cup milk

Preheat oven to 400°. Bring to a boil water, brown sugar and butter. Meanwhile in a bowl mix sugar, flour, salt, baking powder and milk. Pour liquids over the batter. Bake for ½ hour.

Diane Voisine
Fort Kent, Maine

Tester's Note: I cooked this in an 8 x 8-inch greased baking pan, which worked well.

Frozen Lemon Dessert

"This is one of my favorite desserts from childhood. My mother, Virginia, used to make this for special occasions and then watch me like a hawk so that I wouldn't sneak any before our guests had theirs. A few months ago, I had dinner with one of her best friends, Julie. We had this for dessert, and for a moment, we felt "Virginie's" presence."

Preparation Time: 25 minutes

6 to 8 servings

3   egg yolks
½   cup plus 1 tablespoon sugar
¼   cup lemon juice
     Grated rind of ½ lemon
⅛   teaspoon salt (optional)
3   egg whites or ⅓ cup plus 3 tablespoons pasteurized, liquid
       egg whites
1   cup heavy cream, whipped
¾   cup crushed vanilla wafers (about 24 cookies) or graham
       crackers

Beat egg yolks and sugar together. Add lemon juice, rind and salt. Cook mixture in a double boiler until mixture thickens (coats back of spoon without dripping). Cool. Fold in whipped cream. Beat egg whites (or pasteurized egg whites) until stiff and fold into pudding. Line the bottoms of 2 old-fashioned metal ice cube trays with crumbs, pour in pudding, cover and freeze. Serve directly from freezer.

Catherine Maas
Cambridge, Massachusetts

Variations: The pasteurized liquid egg whites worked perfectly in this recipe and avoided any raw egg concerns. Lacking the ice cube trays, a greased 9½-inch springform pan works very well. Fresh strawberries on the side of each serving look and taste delicious!

Stanley Cup Sundaes

"This wonderful sauce recipe was passed down to me by my mother-in-law. My husband always requests this dessert during the Stanley Cup Hockey Finals."

Preparation Time: 10 minutes

Cooking Time: 3 to 4 minutes

4 servings

1	cup sugar
2	tablespoons cocoa
½	teaspoon salt
1	tablespoon flour
½	cup milk
	Lump of butter
½	teaspoon vanilla
	Pecan halves
	Vanilla ice cream

Stir first five ingredients together in a saucepan. Cook over medium heat 3 to 4 minutes to soft boil. Remove from heat, add butter and vanilla and stir. Serve over vanilla ice cream and top with nuts if desired.

Jan LeMessurier Flack
Washington, D.C.

Tester's Note: This is an excellent sauce for ice cream. It is very easy to prepare and very tasty.

Three Fruit Ice

"After a hot day on the beach at my grandparents' home in Antigua, this dessert would refresh me from sunburned lips to sand-burned feet! It can be served elegantly in small bowls with sprigs of mint; or, omitting the egg white, the juice mixture can simply be poured into popsicle forms to serve casually as a snack. My grandmother no longer remembers this, but she always kept the grandchildren happy and healthy with her special treats - one of which was Three Fruit Ice."

Preparation Time: 15 minutes

Cooking Time: 3 minutes

6 servings

1   cup sugar
1   cup water
1   lemon (approximately ¼ cup juice)
1   orange (approximately ½ cup juice)
1   mashed banana
1   egg white, beaten until stiff

In a small saucepan cook the sugar and water until the sugar is completely dissolved. Add all the other ingredients. Pour into a low container (an 8 x 8-inch metal cake pan works well) and put in the freezer. When nearly frozen, beat thoroughly with an electric beater and return to freezer until ready to serve.

Martha Long
Henderson, North Carolina

Note: Pasteurized liquid egg whites (sold in local markets) can substitute for the raw egg white with no change in texture or flavor.

Mom's Pie Crust

Preparation Time: 10 minutes

2 crusts

2   cups flour
1   cup shortening
1   tablespoon salt
4-6 tablespoons cold water

Using a pastry cutter, cut shortening into flour and salt until the mixture resembles peas. Add very cold water, mixing until dough holds together. Do not over mix as this will make your pastry very tough. Roll out with a minimum of extra flour.

J. MacDonald
Warren, Maine

Note: Do not handle the dough with warm hands as this will cause increased toughness.

Chocolate Walnut Pie

"The favorite of the Sudbury Inn!"
Preparation Time: 10 minutes
Baking Time: 50 minutes

8 to 10 servings

1   10-inch pie crust
2   cups chocolate chips
2   cups walnuts
4   eggs
¾   cup sugar
¾   cup light corn syrup
¾   cup butter, melted

Preheat oven to 350°. Place chocolate chips and walnuts in bottom of pie crust. Mix all other ingredients in order and pour over walnuts and chocolate chips. Bake for 50 minutes.

Cheri Thurston (Sudbury Inn)
Bethel, Maine

Hershey Bar Pie

Preparation Time: 20 minutes

8 to 10 servings

1   chocolate crumb pie crust, unbaked
1   8-ounce Hershey bar, broken into pieces
⅓   cup milk
1½ cups miniature marshmallows
2   cups heavy or whipping cream, divided
1   10-ounce can cherry pie filling, chilled

Bake pie crust according to directions, set aside.
Combine chocolate bar pieces, milk and marshmallows
in medium microwave-proof bowl. Microwave on high for
1½ to 2½ minutes or until chocolate is softened. Blend until
mixture is smooth. Cool completely. Whip 1 cup cream until
stiff. Fold into cooled chocolate mixture. Spoon into pie crust.
Garnish with remaining whipped cream. Chill until set for
2 hours. Serve topped with chilled cherry pie filling.

Darla Patheaude
Roxbury, Maine

Graham Cracker Pie

"This is my dad's favorite. We always had it for special occasions, especially Father's Day. You can't beat it for breakfast!"

Preparation Time: 1 hour

Baking Time: 15 minutes

8 to 10 servings

Crust
1½ cups graham cracker crumbs (1 package)
6   tablespoons butter, melted

Filling
3   egg yolks
⅓   cup sugar
¼   teaspoon salt
3   tablespoons cornstarch
1   tablespoon butter, melted
2   cups scalded milk
1   teaspoon vanilla

Meringue
3   egg whites
2   tablespoons powdered sugar
¼   teaspoon vanilla

Preheat oven to 300°. For Crust: Mix together crumbs and butter. Reserve ¼ cup. Press remaining crumbs into 9-inch pie plate. For Filling: In a double boiler, beat egg yolks until pale yellow. Gradually add sugar, salt, cornstarch, and butter. Slowly add 2 cups scalded milk. Stir over boiling water until thick, about 15 minutes. Cool and add vanilla. Pour into crust. For Meringue: Beat egg whites until stiff, gradually adding sugar. Stir in vanilla. Spread meringue on top of filling. Top with reserved crumbs. Bake for 15 minutes. This is best made a day ahead and chilled overnight.

Sally Sewall
South Portland, Maine

Lemon Graham Cracker Crust Pie

"This was one of my mother's recipes that I grew up with."

Preparation Time: 15 to 30 minutes

8 servings

Crust
20   sugar honey graham cracker squares
½   stick margarine or butter, softened
¼   cup sugar

Filling
1   14-ounce can sweetened condensed milk
½   cup lemon juice
      Grated rind of one lemon

Topping
½   cup heavy cream
2   tablespoons confectioners' sugar

Preheat oven to 375°. For Crust: Place graham crackers in
a plastic bag and roll out to fine even crumbs. Pour crumbs into
bowl, add margarine and sugar. Blend well with fingers or fork.
Pour crumb mix into a 9-inch pie plate. Set an 8-inch pie plate on
top and press firmly to make an even layer. Bake for 8 minutes.
For Filling: Blend milk, sugar and lemon rind with a wire whisk.
Pour into cool pie shell. Chill until set. Whip ½ cup cream with
confectioners' sugar until stiff. Spoon onto chilled pie and serve.

Joyce Dexter
Newcastle, Maine

Lemon Meringue Pie

"My mother, Dorothy Skillins, started making this pie in the 1930's. It was always a treat at any meal. It is just as good today."

Preparation Time: 15 minutes

Baking Time: 15 minutes

8 to 10 servings

Pie Shell
1   8-inch graham cracker pie shell

Filling
1   14-ounce can sweetened condensed milk
½   cup lemon juice
1   teaspoon lemon rind (or ¼ teaspoon lemon extract)
2   egg yolks

Topping
2   egg whites
¼   teaspoon cream of tartar
4   tablespoons sugar

Preheat oven to 325°. For Filling: Blend milk, lemon juice, lemon rind or extract and egg yolks. Pour into pie shell. For Topping: Add cream of tartar to egg whites. Beat until almost stiff, just enough to hold a peak. Add sugar gradually, beating until stiff, but not dry. Pile lightly on filling. Bake for 15 minutes or until lightly browned. Cool before serving.

Frances Johnson
Las Cruces, New Mexico

Swedish Apple Pie

"I gave this recipe to the owners of Raymond Apple Orchards. They make the pies to sell at their stand. The recipe is a very easy one, using no lard or butter crust to roll out. The recipe was given to me at an international golf tournament about 8 years ago."

Preparation Time: 30 minutes

Baking Time: 45 minutes

6 to 8 servings

Apple Filling
4   medium apples, sliced
2   tablespoons sugar
1   teaspoon cinnamon
    Dash of nutmeg
    Pinch of salt

Top Crust
¾   cup sugar
¾   cup flour
1   stick butter, melted
1   egg, slightly beaten
½   cup chopped walnuts

Preheat oven to 350°. For Filling: Combine apples with sugar, cinnamon, nutmeg and salt. Pour into a well-greased 9-inch pie plate. For Top Crust: Combine sugar and flour. Add egg to melted butter and mix in with sugar and flour. Add chopped nuts. Spread this batter over apples. Bake for 45 minutes.

Dee P. Dole
Portland, Maine

Cherry Cheese Pie

"A real showy company dessert."

Preparation Time: 20 minutes

Baking Time: 25 minutes

8 to 10 servings

Crust
12-14	graham crackers, crumbled (or 1½ cups packaged crumbs)
½	stick butter, melted
2	tablespoons sugar

Filling
12	ounces cream cheese, room temperature
2	eggs, beaten
½	cup sugar
½	teaspoon vanilla

Topping
1½	cups sour cream
2	tablespoons sugar
2	teaspoons vanilla

Cherry Topping
2	cans Bing cherries
1½	tablespoons cornstarch

Preheat oven to 350°. For Crust: Mix graham cracker crumbs, butter and sugar. Press into a 10-inch glass pie plate. Set aside. For Filling: Beat cream cheese, eggs, sugar and vanilla until smooth and pour into crumb-lined pie plate. Bake for 20 minutes. Remove from oven and immediately spread on topping made of sour cream, sugar and vanilla. Raise oven temperature to 475° and bake pie an additional 5 minutes. Refrigerate immediately. (Pie may be frozen at this point.) For Cherry Topping: Drain and reserve syrup from 2 cans Bing cherries in refrigerator. When pie is cool, arrange cherries on top.

Mix 1½ tablespoons cornstarch with ¼ cup cold cherry juice in saucepan over medium heat. Add ¾ cup more juice and cook until thick and clear. Use a whisk to avoid lumps, being careful not to let the glaze catch. Pour over cherries and allow to cool in refrigerator.

Lynn Goldfarb
Portland, Maine

Note: The glazed pie cannot be frozen as it becomes rubbery.

Dutch Apple Tart

"This recipe was used by my mother who died of Alzheimer's disease in 1990. Born in Pennsylvania, her heritage was Pennsylvania Dutch. I never knew a better cook, nor did I know that most people put a top on apple pie!"

Preparation Time: 30 minutes

Baking Time: 45 to 60 minutes

6 to 8 servings

6 to 7	Macintosh (or other cooking apple), pared and quartered
¾	cup brown sugar
¼	cup flour
½	teaspoon cinnamon
	Salt(optional)
¼	cup evaporated milk or heavy cream
1	9-inch pie crust

Preheat oven to 400°. Place apples cored side down (round side up) in pie crust lined pie plate. Combine sugar, flour, cinnamon, and salt. Sprinkle mixture over apples in pie plate. Pour milk/cream over apples. Bake for 10 minutes; reduce heat to 350° and bake for 45 to 60 minutes or until apples are tender when pricked with fork.

Susan H. Grondin
Raymond, Maine

George Washington Cream Pie

"As children, growing up in Dubuque, Iowa, we looked forward to George Washington's birthday. In anticipation of the coming holiday there was always a school assembly that often included the early demise of the legendary cherry tree and the associated moral lesson about telling the truth. Also eagerly anticipated on the holiday was the George Washington Cream Pie that was produced by many of the mothers in our community. My paternal grandfather was a patriotic state senator who felt that the birthday of the father of our country was a special occasion. Therefore, with our cousins, we were all invited to gather at his house to celebrate. Our mother would see that we were suitably scrubbed, combed and dressed, and we would be loaded into the back seat of the Willys Knight for the trip to our grandparents' house. There we would all be seated at the dining room table, where we would each find a red, white, and blue paper party hat at our place. After a prayer of thanks for the privilege of living in the great United States, grandmother would bring out two of her George Washington Cream Pies."

Preparation Time: 1 hour

Chill: Several hours

8 servings

1   9-inch pie shell, baked

Custard Pie Filling (use ½ recipe for pie; use ½ for another purpose)
3   egg yolks
⅓   cup sugar
¼   teaspoon salt
2½ tablespoons cornstarch
1   tablespoon butter, room temperature
2   cups milk, scalded
1   teaspoon vanilla

Cherry Topping
½ cup sugar
2 tablespoons cornstarch
1 16-ounce can sour red cherries, drained (liquid reserved)
 Cherry liquid plus enough water to make ¾ cup
1 teaspoon lemon juice (or 2 drops almond extract)
 Red food coloring (optional)

For Cream Filling: Beat egg yolks. Gradually beat in sugar, salt, cornstarch and butter. Pour scalded milk over these ingredients and cook, stirring constantly in a double boiler or in a saucepan over very low heat. Remove from heat when thickened and cool. Add 1 teaspoon vanilla. When completely cool, pour into pie shell. For Cherry Topping: Mix sugar and cornstarch in saucepan; gradually blend in cherry liquid and heat, stirring, until boiling. Reduce heat and simmer 5 minutes, stirring occasionally. Off heat mix in lemon juice (or almond extract), cherries and coloring. Cool for 5 minutes. Fill pie shell with ½ custard filling. Add cherry topping and chill in refrigerator for several hours before serving.

Wells Lange
Niwot, Colorado

Note: This pie would also be a perfect choice for the Fourth of July.

Hawaiian Pineapple Pie

Preparation Time: 10 minutes

8 servings

1   graham cracker pie crust
1   3⅛-ounce package sugar-free instant vanilla pudding
2   bananas, sliced
1   20-ounce can crushed pineapple, drained
     Frozen whipped topping
     Crushed walnuts
     Maraschino cherries, cut up

Prepare pudding according to directions using skim milk.
Pour into pie crust. Place sliced bananas on top. Spread pineapple
on top. Cover with frozen whipped topping, crushed walnuts
and a few cherries. Chill.

Nola J. Chaisson
Raymond, Maine

**Note: This is a great dessert for diabetics or those on
low-fat diets.**

Schaum Torte

"In memory of my mother, Virginia Sheehan Maas. Mom made schaum tortes for special dinners when I was a child. This is her mother's recipe. It is the best I have tasted - no restaurant version can compare!"

Preparation Time: 20 minutes

Baking Time: 1 hour

8 servings

Schaum Torte
4   egg whites
1½ cups sugar
1   teaspoon vanilla
1   teaspoon vinegar

Strawberry Topping
1   pint whipping cream
1   teaspoon vanilla
2   boxes fresh strawberries

Preheat oven to 270°. For Tortes: Beat egg whites until stiff and dry. Add sugar, slowly, while beating. Then add vanilla and vinegar. Drop by large tablespoon onto brown paper-lined cookie sheet to make individual tortes (about 2½ to 3" in diameter). Bake for 1 hour or until light brown. Remove from paper immediately. Cool. For Topping: Whip cream until stiff, adding vanilla while beating. Wash and stem strawberries. Slice one box and mix with whipped cream. Spread over individual tortes using whole berries, pointed side up, to decorate.

Patricia Maas Major
Mequon, Wisconsin

Strawberry Cool Whip Pie

"This recipe came from a very dear friend who has since passed away. It makes a wonderful summer dessert."

Preparation Time: 10 minutes

Chill: 2 hours

Two 9-inch pies

1   10-ounce package frozen strawberries, thawed
1   16-ounce container frozen whipped topping
½   teaspoon lemon juice
2   9-inch graham cracker pie shells
    Fresh strawberries for garnish (optional)

Mix strawberries, whipped topping and lemon juice in a large bowl. Divide mixture in half and pour into pie shells. Refrigerate for 2 hours. Garnish with fresh strawberries before serving.

Brenda Sickles
Bangor, Maine

Note: You may substitute strawberries with canned blueberries or canned pineapple.

Strawberry Pie

"This recipe comes from the kitchen of my mother, Virginia Lamphier. She was an excellent cook and her recipes are treasured by her family."

Preparation Time: 10 minutes

Chill: 2 hours

2 9-inch pies (or 16 servings)

1   cup sugar
2   tablespoons cornstarch
2   10-ounce packages frozen strawberries, thawed and drained
     (save juice)
1   3-ounce package strawberry jello
1¾ cups water
2   9-inch pie shells, baked
     Whipped cream or frozen whipped topping

Combine sugar, cornstarch, berry juice, jello and water in a saucepan over medium heat. Stir until dissolved. Cool to room temperature. Arrange berries in bottom of cooked pie shell. Spoon jello mixture over berries. Chill until set, about 2 hours. Top with whipped cream or frozen whipped topping.

Gail Gilmore
Belfast, Maine

Blueberry Peach Pie

Preparation Time: 15 to 30 minutes

Baking Time: 35 to 45 minutes

6 to 8 servings

⅞   cup sugar
5   tablespoons flour
½   teaspoon cinnamon
2   cups fresh blueberries
2   cups fresh peaches, sliced thin
1   tablespoon butter
     Your favorite two crust 9-inch pie pastry

Preheat oven to 375°. Sift dry ingredients into bowl of prepared fruit. Stir well. Pour into 9-inch pie shell. Dot with butter and cover with top layer of pie crust. Brush with milk for a golden brown appearance. Bake for 35 to 45 minutes.

Nancy Bloch
Portland, Maine

Note: This is a pretty filling and looks nice with a latticed top crust.

[handwritten notes: George says "Need to be proud of this recipe!" — Made w/ GF/DF pastry. Aug. 7 '14 for Bethesda family's arrival]

Fruit Topped Cheesecake Pie

Preparation Time: 10 minutes

Chill 2 hours

8 servings

1   baked 9-inch pie shell
1   8-ounce package cream cheese, room temperature
1   cup confectioners' sugar
1   teaspoon vanilla
1   cup whipping cream, whipped
¼   teaspoon almond extract
2   cups thinly sliced fruit in season

Beat together cream cheese, sugar and vanilla until smooth. Fold in almond-flavored whipped cream. Pour into cooked pie shell. Chill, covered, in refrigerator for 2 hours. Just before serving, cover top with fruit.

Donna Oakes
Old Town, Maine

Note: Suggested toppings are cherries, peaches, berries or 1 10-ounce can of fruit pie filling.

Trudy's Turtle Cake

"This cake recipe comes from my husband's mother. It is a sure fire hit. Great with vanilla ice cream or whipped cream!"

Preparation Time: 30 minutes

Baking Time: 35 to 40 minutes

12 to 15 servings

1	chocolate cake mix
1	14-ounce package caramels
½	cup evaporated milk
¾	cup melted butter
1	cup chopped pecans
1	cup chocolate chips

Preheat oven to 350°. Grease and flour 9x13-inch pan. Prepare cake batter according to package directions. Pour half of batter into pan. Bake 15 minutes. Meanwhile, melt caramels, milk and butter together in a small saucepan. Pour over partially baked cake. Sprinkle with nuts and chocolate chips. Top with remaining cake batter and bake an additional 20 to 25 minutes. Cool well before cutting.

Grande Pastry Shop
Portland, Maine

chocolate Gugglehoft

"This cake was always made for family gatherings."

Preparation Time: 25 minutes

Baking Time: 45 minutes to 1 hour

10 to 12 servings

1¾ cups butter, softened
2¼ cups sugar
6   egg yolks
1   cup milk
4¼ cups flour, sifted and divided
¼   teaspoon grated lemon rind
1   teaspoon baking powder
6   egg whites, stiffly beaten
4   tablespoons cocoa
4-5 tablespoons water
2   tablespoons sugar

Preheat oven to 325°. Beat butter until creamy. Add sugar, egg yolks, milk, 2⅛ cups sifted flour, and lemon rind. Stir until fluffy. Combine baking powder with remaining flour. Add to mixture. Fold in egg whites. Divide batter into 2 parts. Stir cocoa with water and 2 tablespoons sugar. Add to one half of the batter. In a deep greased ring mold, put a layer of white batter and then a layer of chocolate batter. Repeat. Bake 45 minutes to 1 hour.

Marcia Kay
Bethesda, Maryland

Sour Cream Chocolate Cake

Preparation Time: 30 minutes

Baking Time: 35 to 45 minutes

10 to 12 servings

Cake
¼   cup butter, softened
2   eggs
2   cups sugar
2   cups flour
1¼ teaspoons baking soda
1   teaspoon salt
½   teaspoon baking powder
1   cup water
1   teaspoon vanilla extract
¾   cup sour cream
4   ounces unsweetened chocolate, melted

Frosting
⅓   cup butter, softened
3   ounces unsweetened chocolate, melted
3   cups confectioners' sugar
2   teaspoons vanilla extract
½   cup sour cream

Preheat oven to 350°. For Cake: Mix all ingredients in large bowl of electric mixer. Beat ½ minute on low, then 3 minutes on high. Batter is very creamy and smooth. Pour into 2 greased and floured 9-inch cake pans. Bake 35 to 45 minutes. Cool on rack. For Frosting: Mix all ingredients together until smooth. Frost cake when cool.

Patsy Leavitt
Buxton, Maine

Note: A great chocolate cake that is good for special occasions.

Raspberry Chocolate Truffle Cake

Preparation Time: 30 to 45 minutes

Baking Time: 20 to 25 minutes

8 servings

Chocolate Biscuit
4   eggs, separated
⅔   cup sugar, divided
¼   cup flour
2   tablespoons cocoa
½   tablespoon cornstarch
2   ounces butter, melted

Truffle Mixture
8   ounces semisweet chocolate
1½ cups whipping cream
¼   cup sugar
½   cup raspberries
¼   cup raspberry jam
2   tablespoons fruit liqueur (preferably raspberry or kirsch)
     Confectioners' sugar

Preheat oven to 350° For Biscuit: Beat egg yolks and ⅓ cup sugar until light lemon color. In clean bowl, beat egg whites and ⅓ cup sugar until stiff. Carefully fold into yolk mixture. Sift flour, cocoa and cornstarch and fold into egg mixture. Add melted butter and mix gently. Pour into greased and floured 8-inch springform pan. Bake 20 to 25 minutes, or until toothpick comes out clean. Cool on rack. For Truffle Mixture: Melt chocolate and stir until smooth. In clean bowl beat whipping cream and sugar until stiff. Gently fold into chocolate. Set aside. Release side of springform pan and carefully slice cake in half to form 2 layers. Remove upper half. Return bottom layer to pan and replace side of pan to hold. Brush bottom layer of cake with liqueur and then jam. Place raspberries over top. Pour truffle mixture over top of raspberries. Crumble other cake layer over truffle. Sprinkle with confectioners' sugar.

Judy Kane
Falmouth, Maine

Note: Easy, delicious - especially the leftovers - if there are any!

chocolate Syrup cake

Preparation Time: 10 minutes

Baking Time: 50 to 60 minutes

10 to 12 servings

1   package yellow cake mix
1   3⅛-ounce package butterscotch instant pudding mix
½   cup oil
1   teaspoon vanilla extract
4   eggs
1   cup hot water
1   cup chocolate syrup

Preheat oven to 350°. Mix all ingredients together, except syrup. Put ¾ batter into greased bundt pan. Add chocolate syrup to remaining cake batter. Mix well. Pour on top of batter in pan. Do not mix. Bake 50 to 60 minutes.

Dorothy Crandell
Scarborough, Maine

chocolate cake

"My mother would get up at 5:00 AM and whip up 24 cupcakes to go in the lunch boxes of seven children or for the child who remembered-always at the last minute-the school party for which he or she had blithely promised Mom's great cupcakes! This is my grandmother's wartime "eggless, milkless" cake recipe."

Preparation Time: 15 minutes

Baking Time: Cupcakes: 15 minutes; Cake: 25 to 30 minutes

24 cupcakes, 1 tube cake or 1 13x9-inch cake

Cake
3   cups flour
8   tablespoons cocoa powder
2   teaspoons instant coffee
2   teaspoons baking soda
1   teaspoon salt
2   cups sugar
½   cup shortening
2   tablespoons vinegar
2   teaspoons vanilla
2   cups water

Raspberry Fluff Frosting (optional)
1   large egg white
1   cup sugar
1   cup fresh raspberries (or strawberries)

Preheat oven to 350°. For Cake: Measure flour, cocoa, instant coffee, baking soda and salt into sifter. Cream sugar and shortening in mixing bowl. Stir in vinegar and vanilla. Sift in dry ingredients, adding alternately with water and beating with electric mixer until smooth. Bake cupcakes for 15 minutes or cake for 25 to 30 minutes. For Topping: Beat egg white until part-way stiff, then gradually add sugar and raspberries (strawberries) while continuing to beat on high speed until fluff is stiff.

Liz Weaver
Cape Elizabeth, Maine

Note: Cakes may also be topped with vanilla frosting.

Black Bottom Cupcakes

"Today I stand at my mother's sink doing the dishes and looking out over the same view of harbor and islands she enjoyed. I have become my mother after all! This recipe was one she used to make and send to me at Westbrook Junior College, packed in waxed paper in a shoe box. My dormmates always knew about those goodie packages from home. I was unusually popular on those mail days. Thank you, Mama, for your thoughtfulness and your example."

Preparation Time: 20 minutes

Baking Time: 30 minutes

30 cupcakes

Cheese Topping
1	8-ounce package cream cheese, softened
⅛	teaspoon salt
1	egg, unbeaten
⅓	cup sugar
8	ounces chocolate bits
½	cup chopped pecans (optional)

Chocolate Cake
2¼	cups flour
1⅔	cups sugar
⅓	cup cocoa
1½	teaspoons baking soda
¾	teaspoon salt
1½	cups cold water
½	cup oil
1½	teaspoons vinegar
1	teaspoon vanilla extract

Preheat oven to 350°. For Cheese Topping: Blend first four ingredients. Add chocolate bits and nuts (if desired). Set aside. For Cakes: Sift flour, sugar, cocoa, soda and salt into bowl. Make a hole in center of sifted ingredients and put in water, oil, vinegar, and vanilla. Mix well. Fill to ⅔ medium paper muffin liners. Top, in center, with 1 tablespoon cheese mixture. Bake for about 30 minutes.

Sheila Thomas Hill
Spruce Head, Maine

Swiss Apple Dessert Pancakes

"This recipe is from a tiny town in the Swiss Alps."

Preparation Time: 20 minutes
6 to 8 pancakes

Apple Topping
1½ cups apples, cored, peeled, cut in chunks
1   tablespoon unsalted butter
     Sugar
     Cinnamon

Pancakes
1½ cups flour
½   teaspoon baking powder
½   teaspoon salt
2   eggs, medium or large
2   cups milk
     Butter, unsalted (for frying)
     Confectioners' sugar

For Apple Topping: Sauté prepared apples in butter. Sprinkle with cinnamon and sugar. Do not over cook. Keep firm. For Pancakes: Sift flour, baking powder, and salt together. Add eggs, beaten in milk. Stir until batter is perfectly smooth. Heat 8-inch fry pan. Cover sides and bottom with butter. Pour enough batter just to cover bottom of pan. Cook until brown around edges and flip to other side. Remove to warm oven until all pancakes are cooked. Divide apple mixture among pancakes, spreading on top of each. Roll and sprinkle with confectioners' sugar.

Vera Lagomarsino
Cape Elizabeth, Maine

Optional: Add raisins and pecans to apple mixture. Substitute berries for apples. Also delicious when served with ice cream or whipped cream.

Gobs

"This is the western Pennsylvania version of Whoopie Pies—these cookies are smaller, less chocolatey, not so sweet, and the filling is smooth rather than gritty. As a transplanted Pennsylvanian, maybe I'm just prejudiced, but in our house, we've always thought that Gobs taste better than Whoopie Pies. My dear aunt Ida Carlucci of Charleroi, Pennsylvania, now in her 80's and memory-impaired, used to make these cookies often when I was a child there; this is her recipe, which I have cherished for 35 years."

Preparation Time: 1½ hours

Baking Time: 5 minutes

3 dozen

Cakes
4	cups flour
1	teaspoon salt
½	cup cocoa
2	teaspoons baking soda
½	teaspoon baking powder
2	cups sugar
½	cup margarine or butter, softened
2	eggs
1	cup buttermilk
1	teaspoon vanilla
¾	cup boiling water

Filling
5	tablespoons flour
1	cup milk
1	cup powdered sugar
½	cup margarine or butter, softened
1	teaspoon vanilla
½	cup shortening or butter, softened

Preheat oven to 450°. For Filling: Mix in saucepan off heat 5 tablespoons flour and 1 cup milk. Place over medium heat. Boil until thick, stirring constantly. Cover and let cool completely away from heat. Make cakes while this mixture cools. For Cakes: Sift together flour, salt and cocoa, baking soda and baking powder. Cream together sugar, margarine or butter. Beat in eggs. Beat in buttermilk, vanilla, and boiling water. Add dry ingredients. Mix well. Drop by rounded teaspoonfuls onto ungreased cookie sheets. Bake for 5 minutes. Remove from cookie sheets. Cool. Finish the filling: Beat together the remaining filling ingredients. Add cooled milk and flour mixture. Beat altogether with electric mixer until smooth and fluffy. Spread filling between 2 cakes and sandwich them together.

Donna Marchinetti
Portland, Maine

Pumpkin Whoopie Pies

Preparation Time: 20 minutes

Baking Time: 13 minutes per cookie sheet

24 filled pies

Pies
1   16-ounce can pumpkin
2   cups sugar
1   cup vegetable oil
2   eggs, beaten
4   cups flour
4   teaspoons baking powder
2   teaspoons cinnamon
1   teaspoon salt
1   teaspoon nutmeg
2   teaspoons baking soda
2   teaspoons milk

Filling
1   cup shortening
1   stick butter or margarine
2   teaspoons vanilla extract
1   7½-ounce jar Marshmallow Fluff
2   teaspoons milk
3⅓ cups confectioners' sugar

Preheat oven to 375°. For Pies: Mix all ingredients together either by hand or electric mixer until well moistened. Place by teaspoonful on ungreased cookie sheets or baking stone. You should get 48 single pies. Bake for 13 minutes. Remove from cookie sheets and cool on wire racks. For Filling: Combine all ingredients until smooth. Spread filling between two pies and sandwich together.

Kathy Dow
Owl's Head, Maine

Note: This recipe was given to me a few years ago. They are absolutely the best treats that I have ever made. They are a hit with everyone. They keep well, staying very moist. Usually they're not around long enough for that to be a problem, though!

Old Fashioned Pound Cake

"This is the ultimate comfort food, which always reminds me of home and family. My mom taught me to bake using this recipe. Enjoy!"

Preparation Time: 20 minutes

Baking Time: 1 hour

10 to 12 servings

Cake

2	sticks butter, softened
2	sticks margarine, softened
1	16-ounce box powdered sugar
6	eggs
3	cups sifted flour
2	tablespoons orange juice
1	tablespoon vanilla

Cream Cheese Frosting

1	8-ounce package cream cheese, softened
4	tablespoons butter, softened
1	16-ounce box powdered sugar
1	teaspoon vanilla

Preheat oven to 350°. For Cake: Cream butter, margarine and sugar until smooth and lemon colored. Add eggs one at a time. Gradually add flour and blend. Add orange juice and vanilla. Bake in greased and floured tube pan for 1 hour. For Frosting: Blend all ingredients until smooth. Frost cake when cool.

Susan Braziel
Cape Elizabeth, Maine

Easy Sponge Cake

"Really great with a cup of tea and conversation with a friend."

Preparation Time: 15 minutes

Baking Time: 40 minutes

2 small loaves

2	eggs
1	cup sugar
1	cup flour
1	teaspoon baking powder
½	teaspoon salt
½	cup hot milk
2	tablespoons melted margarine or butter
1	teaspoon lemon extract

Preheat oven to 350°. Beat eggs until fluffy. Add sugar. Sift flour with baking powder and salt. Add to egg mixture. Gradually add milk, margarine or butter and lemon extract. Pour into 2 3x5-inch mini loaf pans that have been greased and floured. Bake about 40 minutes. Let rest in pans for 5 minutes before removing to rack to cool.

Evelyn H. Towne
Waterville, Maine

Passover Sponge Cake

"My mother used to make one to two of these cakes a day during Passover. Often I would wake up at 6:00 AM to the sound of the Mixmaster. This moist cake was always a big hit and my mother gave many of them away. Now that my mother is gone, I am the keeper of the recipe and make it for the Passover Seders with the family."

Preparation Time: 25 minutes

Baking Time: 1 hour 10 minutes

8 to 10 servings

⅓   cup cake meal (or cake flour)
⅓   cup potato starch
9   eggs, separated
1½ cups sugar, divided
`   Grated rind of 1 lemon
     Nuts (optional)

Preheat oven to 325°. Mix cake flour and potato starch. Beat egg whites until stiff. Add ½ cup of the sugar and beat for 1 to 2 minutes. Set aside. Beat egg yolks with remaining sugar until light and lemon colored. Add lemon rind and mix thoroughly. Add cake flour and starch. Mix. If desired, nuts may be added here. Add mixture to egg whites and bake in ungreased aluminum tube pan, with removable ring and bottom. (Do not use dark coated pan.) Bake for 1 hour. Cool upside down in pan for an hour before removing.

Sheila Levine
Arlington, Virginia

Tester's Note: This is not a sweet cake, but is light textured and flavorful. I didn't have a lemon so I used an orange. Either lemon or orange works well. I glazed my cake with an orange glaze.

Norwegian Gold Cake

"When my four brothers and sisters and I were growing up, we got to choose our birthday dinner menu, including our choice of cake. Despite the lack of icing, the Norwegian Gold Cake was a frequent selection!"

Preparation Time: 20 minutes

Baking Time: 1 hour

14 slices

2   sticks butter, softened
1½ cups flour
5   eggs
1⅓ cups sugar
1¼ teaspoons baking powder
¼   teaspoon salt
2   teaspoons almond extract
1   cup plain breadcrumbs (to coat cake pan)

Preheat oven to 325°. Cream butter and flour for 5 minutes. Complete the whole 5 minutes as this is the key to a light textured, successful cake. Then add 1 egg at a time. Beat until well blended. Sift together sugar, baking powder, and salt. Add to butter mixture. Add almond extract. Grease a tube pan with butter. Put in bread crumbs and roll to coat pan with an even thin layer. Discard excess crumbs. Pour in batter. Bake for approximately 1 hour or until cake springs back to light touch.

Constance McCabe
Pownal, Maine

Loaf Cake with Raisins

Preparation Time: 10 minutes
Baking Time: 1 hour

12 servings

1   cup sugar
½   cup butter, softened
½   teaspoon baking powder
1½ cups sifted flour
2   eggs
½   cup milk
1   cup raisins, floured

Preheat oven to 350°. Cream sugar and butter. Add eggs, one at a time, and beat well. Add milk, flour, baking powder and raisins. Bake for 1 hour in greased loaf pan.

Lynn Goldfarb
Portland, Maine

Note: Great to keep in the freezer to take as a gift or to serve to unexpected guests. Good with blueberries, too!

Lemon Sauce

Preparation Time: 10 minutes

4 servings

1   rounded teaspoon cornstarch
½   cup sugar
1   cup boiling water
2   tablespoons butter
1   teaspoon lemon extract
¼   teaspoon nutmeg
¼   teaspoon salt

Mix cornstarch and sugar in a small saucepan. Add hot water and cook over medium heat until thickened, stirring constantly for 4 to 5 minutes. Remove from heat and add butter. Stir until melted. Add remaining ingredients and serve over cake or pudding, hot or cold.

Erna Smith
Lisbon Falls, Maine

white cake

*"My husband's father lived with us for nearly nine years.
This cake, topped with a chocolate frosting, was his favorite.
It originated with my great-grandmother, but is known in our
house as 'Grampa's Birthday Cake'."*

Preparation Time: 25 minutes

Baking Time: 25 to 30 minutes

12 servings

2	cups pre-sifted flour
1½	cups sugar
½	teaspoon salt
½	cup shortening
1	cup milk
1	teaspoon vanilla
2	eggs
3	teaspoons baking powder
	Chocolate frosting

Preheat oven to 350°. Measure flour, sugar and salt into sifter.
Measure shortening, milk and vanilla into mixing bowl. Add dry
ingredients from sifter. Beat 2 minutes with electric mixer or until
smooth. Add eggs and baking soda. Beat 2 minutes more until
smooth. Pour into 2 greased and floured 13x9x2-inch pans.
Bake 25 to 30 minutes. Top with chocolate frosting.

*Liz Weaver
Cape Elizabeth, Maine*

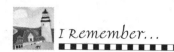

Brownie Schrumpf's Angel Gingerbread

"First made by Nellie Brown, Brownie and Doris' mother, on the farm in Readfield Depot, Maine."

Preparation Time: 15 minutes

Baking Time: 35 to 40 minutes

9 servings

½	cup sugar
½	cup molasses
½	cup shortening, melted
1	egg, beaten
1½	cups flour
1	teaspoon baking soda
¼	teaspoon salt
½	teaspoon ginger
½	teaspoon cinnamon
½	cup boiling water

Preheat oven to 350°. Beat sugar, molasses and shortening. Sift dry ingredients together. Add to sugar mixture. Add ½ cup boiling water. Mix well. Fold into 8x8-inch pan. Bake for 35 to 40 minutes.

Doris Brown Dow (Brownie's sister)
Winthrop, Maine

Note: Great taste served with hot applesauce.

Sponge Gingerbread

"A favorite recipe that my grandmother used to make for us."

Preparation Time: 10 minutes

Baking Time: 25 to 30 minutes

9 servings

1	cup sugar
½	cup molasses
½	cup shortening, melted
1	egg
1	teaspoon baking soda
1	teaspoon cinnamon
1½	cups sifted flour
1	cup boiling water

Preheat oven to 350°. Beat first seven ingredients together.
Add 1 cup boiling water and beat well. Mixture will be thin.
Pour into greased 9-inch square pan. Bake for 25 to 30 minutes.

Cindy Dodge
Freeport, Maine

Tester's Note: Smelled great cooking! Lovely served with fresh whipped cream.

Muster Gingerbread

"This recipe gets its name from having been served on muster days in southern Maine. It was passed down from the late 1700's by my ancestor, Sally Emery Hodsdon, of Poland, Maine. The measurements have been standardized."

Preparation Time: 10 to 15 minutes

Baking Time: 20 minutes

2 dozen servings

⅓   cup shortening
⅓   cup brown sugar
1   egg, beaten
½   cup molasses
1¾ cups flour
2   teaspoons ginger
½   teaspoon cinnamon
¾   teaspoon salt
½   teaspoon soda

Preheat oven to 350°. Cream shortening, adding sugar gradually. Add egg and molasses. Beat out any lumps. Mix flour and spices in small bowl with salt and soda. Stir into mixture and blend well. Spread evenly in a 13x9x2-inch greased pan. Put flour on your hand to press evenly. Bake for 20 minutes, or until edges begin to brown. Cut in squares.

Beverly Boardman
Bangor, Maine

Note: This bar-like cake has a gingersnap flavor and is especially good with a glass of milk.

cheese cake

Preparation Time: 20 minutes

Baking Time: 50 to 55 minutes

10 to 12 servings

Crust
1¼ cups graham cracker crumbs
¼   cup sugar
⅓   cup melted butter or margarine

Cheese Filling
3   eggs
1   cup sugar
1   pound cream cheese, softened
1   teaspoon almond extract
2   teaspoons vanilla extract
3   cups sour cream
1   pint fresh strawberries

Preheat oven to 375°. For Crust: Mix graham cracker crumbs with sugar and margarine or butter. Press into 9-inch spring form pan. For Cheese Filling: Beat eggs and sugar until thick. Add cream cheese and beat until smooth. Add almond and vanilla extracts. Blend in sour cream. Pour filling into spring form pan lined with graham cracker crumbs. Bake for 50 to 55 minutes. Turn off oven and let cheese cake cool in the oven with the door open. This will keep the cake from cracking. Refrigerate. Best made a day ahead. Halve strawberries and place on top just before serving.

Barbara Schenkel
Cape Elizabeth, Maine

Note: This looks beautiful, tastes wonderful and is incredibly easy to make.

Peanut Butter Cheesecake

"This recipe was my mother's. We lost her to Alzheimer's on January 1, 1995. This was by far her favorite recipe. She grew up a chocolate lover, but somewhere along the line switched to peanut butter. It took me a while to acquire a taste for this as it is quite rich, but very delicious. At our family get-togethers, our out-of-state families always looked forward to this cheesecake. At our first gathering after my mother passed away, I made it to bring to the reunion. Needless to say, she was there with us in spirit and there were a few tears brought on by her cheesecake."

Preparation Time: 30 minutes

Chill: 2 to 3 hours

10 to 12 servings

⅓	cup margarine or butter
⅔	cup graham cracker crumbs, divided
¾	cup chopped peanuts, divided
1	12-ounce package cream cheese, softened
⅔	cup peanut butter
1	14-ounce can sweetened condensed milk
⅓	cup lemon juice
1	teaspoon vanilla extract
8	ounces frozen whipped topping

In a small pan, melt margarine or butter. Stir in graham cracker crumbs and peanuts, reserving 2 tablespoons of each for garnish. Press mixture on bottom of greased 9-inch spring form pan. Chill in refrigerator while preparing filling. In large bowl beat cream cheese and peanut butter until fluffy. Add condensed milk and beat until smooth. Stir in lemon juice and vanilla. Fold in frozen whipped topping. Turn into prepared pan and garnish with reserved crumbs and peanuts. Chill 2 to 3 hours. Keep refrigerated.

Dawn A. Leavitt for Leona Locklin Pierce
Kezar Falls, Maine

Ricotta Cheese Cake

Preparation Time: 30 minutes

Baking Time: 1 hour

8 servings

Crust
1   cup confectioners' sugar
½   cup butter, softened
1⅓ cups chopped hazelnuts

Cheese Filling
1   pound ricotta cheese
2   8-ounce packages cream cheese, softened
1   cup sugar
2   egg whites
½   teaspoon lemon juice
½   teaspoon vanilla extract
3   tablespoons butter, melted
1   pint sour cream

Fruit Topping
    Fresh or frozen raspberries

Preheat oven to 325°. For Crust: Combine confectioners' sugar, butter and hazelnuts. Press into 8-inch or 10-inch springform pan. Set aside. For Cheese Filling: Cream ricotta cheese, cream cheese, sugar and egg whites. Add lemon juice and vanilla. Blend until very smooth. Add melted butter and sour cream. Pour cheese mixture into crust. Set springform pan onto a cookie sheet before placing in oven. Bake for 1 hour. Turn off oven and let cake stand in oven for 2 hours. Serve with fresh or frozen raspberries.

Tonia Nadzo Medd
Peaks Island, Maine

Kuchen

"This is a traditional Swiss recipe. When I was teaching 2nd grade in 1978, I became friends with a Swiss family studying in New York for a year. Dorette made this dessert for me the first night I visited them. She made it with figs. Over the year, I had it with many different combinations of fruit. This past fall, 1998, I visited her in Geneva and again had the Kuchen for dessert. We finished it the next morning for breakfast without the sour cream topping. It is always delicious."

Preparation Time: 20 minutes

Baking Time: 35 to 40 minutes

8 to 10 servings

1½ cups flour, divided
½   teaspoon salt, divided
½   cup butter
⅓   cup sour cream, divided
4   cups fruit
3   egg yolks, beaten
1   cup sugar
     Nutmeg (optional)
     Additional sour cream (optional)

Preheat oven to 375°. Mix 1¼ cups flour and ¼ teaspoon salt. Cut in butter until pieces are pea sized. Stir in 2 tablespoons sour cream. Press mixture into 9x9-inch baking dish or pie plate. Bake for 20 minutes. Spread fruit, decoratively, on baked shell. Mix ¼ cup flour, ¼ teaspoon salt, remaining sour cream, egg yolks and sugar. Pour over fruit. Bake for 35 to 40 minutes, or until firm. Cool. Serve with sour cream sprinkled with nutmeg, if desired.

Gail Dransfield
Cape Elizabeth, Maine

Note: Fruit suggestions: plums, apples with cranberries, figs, pears, or peaches.

Orange Fruit Cake

"This recipe was made by my grandmother. I have made it yearly for 42 years and now my grandchildren are enjoying it with the capable hands of my children doing the baking."

Preparation Time: 40 minutes

Baking Time: 2 hours + 5 minutes or longer

20 to 24 slices

Cake
1½ cups sugar
¾ cup shortening
3 eggs
1½ teaspoons baking soda
  Pinch of salt
1 cup sour milk or buttermilk
3 cups flour
1 teaspoon vanilla extract
½ cup raisins
½ cup chopped dates
1 cup chopped nuts
1 pound candied fruit

Sauce
  Juice of 1 orange
¼ cup sugar

Preheat oven to 350°. For Cake: Cream sugar and shortening. Add eggs, baking soda, salt, sour milk or buttermilk, flour and vanilla. Blend well. Fold in raisins, dates, nuts and candied fruit. Pour into greased and floured Bundt or angel food cake pan. Bake for 20 minutes. Reduce heat to 200° and bake for additional 1¾ hours or more. Keep testing with a toothpick until it comes out clean. For Sauce: While cake is cooking, heat orange juice and sugar until well blended and hot. Cool cake in pan and, while still warm, pour on orange sauce.

Barbara Curtis
Belfast, Maine

Coffee Fruit Cake

Preparation Time: 25 minutes

Baking Time: 1½ hours or longer

2 loaves, 20 to 24 servings

1 pound raisins (2½ cups)
1½ cups coffee
1½ cups sugar
½ cup shortening
2 eggs
2½ cups flour
1 teaspoon baking powder
½ teaspoon salt
1 teaspoon cinnamon
½ teaspoon cloves
½ teaspoon allspice
½ cup chopped walnuts
1 cup chopped dates
1 8-ounce jar candied fruit

Preheat oven to 350°. Cook together in a large saucepan, raisins, coffee and sugar. Simmer for 5 minutes. Cool. Then add and mix, shortening, eggs, flour, baking powder, salt, spices, nuts, dates and candied fruit. Pour into 2 greased and floured 8½x4½x4½-inch loaf pans and bake for 30 minutes. Reduce heat to 300° and bake an hour longer, or until toothpick comes out clean.

Christine M. Munsey
Wiscasset, Maine

Party Cake

"I have served this at our Senior Club meetings several times."

Preparation Time: 40 minutes

Baking Time: 15 to 20 minutes

24 servings

1	yellow cake mix
1	package instant yellow pudding
1	cup milk
1	8-ounce package cream cheese, softened
1	9-ounce container frozen whipped topping
1	20-ounce can crushed pineapple, drained several hours
1	cup coconut
1	cup chopped nuts
1	10-ounce jar cherries, drained

Preheat oven to 350°. Prepare cake mix as directed. Bake in greased jelly roll pan 15 to 20 minutes. Cool cake. Dissolve pudding mix in milk and set aside. Cream the cream cheese. Add whipped topping and beat. Add pudding and beat until the consistency of whipped cream. Spread over cool cake. Spread pineapple over top. Sprinkle with coconut, nuts and cherries.

Althea Sage
Howland, Maine

Banana Cake

Preparation Time: 10 minutes

Baking Time: 50 minutes

8 to 10 servings

½ cup butter, room temperature
½-1 cup sugar, depending on taste
2 tablespoons light brown sugar
1 egg, beaten
½ teaspoon almond extract
1¾ cups flour
1 teaspoon baking soda
1 teaspoon baking powder
⅔ teaspoon salt
⅔ teaspoon cider vinegar
⅔ cup evaporated milk
½ cup chopped nuts
1⅓ cups ripe mashed bananas (3 medium)

Preheat oven to 350°. Cream sugars with butter. Add egg mixed with almond extract. Sift flour with baking powder, soda and salt. Add to sugar mixture. Add evaporated milk mixed with vinegar. Blend well. Add nuts and bananas. Beat while singing two stanzas of "Annie Laurie." Bake in greased 9¼x5¼-inch loaf pan for about 50 minutes.

Lucille S. Clark
Cumberland Foreside, Maine

Note: The singing is the fun part and you can choose your own ethnic music!

Apple cake

Preparation Time: 25 minutes

Baking Time: 40 minutes

8 servings

1   cup sugar
2   tablespoons shortening
1   egg
1   teaspoon vanilla
1   cup flour
1   teaspoon salt
1   teaspoon cinnamon
1   teaspoon nutmeg
1   teaspoon baking soda (scant)
3   cups diced, peeled (or unpeeled) apples
½   cup chopped walnuts

Preheat oven to 350°. Cream together shortening and sugar.
Add egg and vanilla. Sift dry ingredients together over chopped
apples and walnuts. Toss to coat. Mix with egg mixture and pour
into greased and floured 7½x11½-inch pan. Bake 40 minutes.

Hope Stacey
Parsonsfield, Maine

**Note: This is most delicious when served warm with vanilla ice
cream, but it may also be served plain or with whipped cream.**

Applesauce Cake

Preparation Time: 20 minutes

Baking Time: 45 minutes

2 loaves

2	cups flour
1	teaspoon baking soda
1	teaspoon cinnamon
½	teaspoon cloves
½	teaspoon allspice (optional)
⅛	teaspoon salt
1	cup sugar
½	cup margarine
1	teaspoon vanilla
1	cup unsweetened applesauce (preferably homemade)

Preheat oven to 350°. Measure all dry ingredients into a bowl or sifter and set aside. Cream margarine and sugar together. Add applesauce and vanilla to this mixture. Stir in dry ingredients. Divide equally into 2 9¼x5¼-inch greased loaf pans. Bake for 45 minutes or until toothpick comes out clean.

Liz Weaver
Cape Elizabeth, Maine

Mama's Spice Cake

"Because this recipe has no eggs and only ½ cup shortening, it was considered an economical dessert during World War II and the Depression years before that."

Preparation Time: 10 minutes

Baking Time: 35 minutes

9 servings

1   cup sour milk or buttermilk
1   teaspoon baking soda
½   cup shortening, melted
1   cup sugar
1   teaspoon cinnamon
¼   teaspoon cloves
1   teaspoon allspice
2   cups flour
     Salt (optional)
     Raisins (amount to taste)

Preheat oven to 350°. Combine sour milk (buttermilk), baking soda and set aside. Mix melted shortening and sugar together. Sift together cinnamon, cloves, allspice, dash salt (if desired) and flour. Add to shortening mixture, alternating with milk. Add raisins. Pour into greased and floured 9-inch round cake pan. Bake for 30 to 35 minutes.

Carol Reidy
Biddeford, Maine

Note: Make sour milk by combining 1 cup milk with 1 tablespoon vinegar.

chocolate zucchini cake

Preparation Time: 30 minutes

Baking Time: 40 to 50 minutes

36 servings

1¾ cups sugar
½ cup margarine or butter
½ cup vegetable oil
2 large eggs
1 teaspoon vanilla
½ cup buttermilk
2½ cups all-purpose flour
1 teaspoon cinnamon
½ teaspoon salt
1 teaspoon baking soda
1 teaspoon baking powder
3 tablespoons unsweetened cocoa powder
2 cups firmly packed, grated, unpeeled zucchini
½ cup semisweet chocolate bits
½ cup chopped walnuts

Preheat oven to 325°. In large mixing bowl, cream together sugar, butter, oil, eggs, vanilla and buttermilk. Mix flour, cinnamon, salt, baking soda, baking powder and cocoa. Add to creamed mixture. Stir in zucchini. Pour into greased and floured 9x13x2-inch pan. Sprinkle on chocolate bits and nuts. Bake 40 to 50 minutes or until toothpick inserted near center comes out clean.

The Lamp (Alzheimer's Residential Care Facility)
Lisbon, Maine

Melt In Your Mouth Blueberry Cake

"When I was growing up, my mother used to make blueberry cake every August using wild Maine blueberries. I now carry on the tradition by making it every summer, too. This is my favorite recipe."

Preparation Time: 15 minutes

Baking Time: 50 to 60 minutes

9 servings

2   eggs, separated
1   cup sugar, divided
¼   teaspoon salt
½   cup shortening
1½ cups sifted flour
1   teaspoon baking powder
⅓   cup milk
1½ cups fresh Maine blueberries
1   teaspoon vanilla extract

Preheat oven to 350°. Beat egg whites until stiff in a small glass bowl. Add about ¼ cup sugar to keep them stiff. Cream shortening and add salt and vanilla. Add remaining sugar gradually. Add unbeaten egg yolks and beat until light and creamy. Add dry ingredients, alternating with milk. Fold in beaten whites. Fold in fresh berries lightly floured. Turn into greased 8x8-inch pan and sprinkle top with sugar. Bake for 50 to 60 minutes.

The Honorable Susan M. Collins, U.S. Senator
Bangor, Maine

Check Inge's Recipe - if same, go for it; if not, make Inge's - same as Inge's, except I have it been adding the vanilla Aug 6 '11

Carrot Cake with Cream Cheese Icing

"This recipe was found in a supplement to 'Country America Magazine'. It was called 'Collin Raye's Carrot Cake.' Raye got this recipe from a fan who presented him with the cake after a performance. I make this cake for all bake sales and functions in the facility in which I work, a residential care unit for patients with Alzheimer's disease and other dementias in Rumford, Maine."

Preparation Time: 30 to 40 minutes

Baking Time: 30 to 35 minutes

24 servings

Cake
2	cups flour
2	cups sugar
1	tablespoon baking powder
1	teaspoon cinnamon
½	teaspoon salt
½	teaspoon nutmeg
3	cups finely shredded carrot
1	cup cooking oil
1	cup finely chopped walnuts
4	eggs

Frosting
¼	cup butter or margarine, softened
¼	cup shortening
12	ounces cream cheese, softened
1	tablespoon vanilla extract
1½	cups sifted confectioners' sugar
2	tablespoons milk (optional)

Preheat oven to 350°. For Cake: Combine flour, sugar, baking powder, cinnamon, salt and nutmeg. Add carrot, cooking oil and nuts. Stir until combined. Add eggs and mix well. Spread evenly in greased 9x13x2-inch pan. Bake 30 to 35 minutes, or until top springs back when lightly touched. Cool on wire rack.

For Frosting: In medium bowl, stir together butter or margarine, shortening, cream cheese and vanilla. Add powdered sugar and stir until smooth. Add enough milk to make good spreading consistency. Frost cool cake. Refrigerate leftovers.

Charlotte Rose
Byron, Maine

Pistachio cake

Preparation Time: 15 minutes

Baking Time: 1 hour

16 to 20 servings

1   white cake mix
2   3⅛-ounce packages instant pistachio pudding mix
4   eggs
1   8-ounce bottle club soda
½   cup vegetable oil
1   teaspoon almond extract
⅓   cup chopped nuts
½   cup chopped cherries
    Confectioners' sugar

Preheat oven to 350°. Mix cake mix, pudding, eggs, club soda, oil and almond extract in large electric mixer bowl. Beat for 4 minutes. Fold in nuts and cherries. Pour batter into greased and floured bundt pan. Bake for 1 hour. Cool on wire rack. Sprinkle with confectioners' sugar when cool.

Debbie Taylor
Hampden, Maine

Note: I make this for special occasions, especially Christmas because of the red and green colors.

Almond Date Squares

Preparation Time: 25 minutes

Baking Time: 30 minutes

36 squares

½   cup butter or margarine
½   cup white sugar
2   egg yolks
1½ cups all-purpose flour
1   teaspoon baking powder
1   teaspoon vanilla
1   cup chopped dates
½   cup water
2   egg whites
1   cup brown sugar
½   cup slivered almonds

Preheat oven to 350°. Bottom layer: Mix first six ingredients together well. Press into a greased 9x9-inch pan. Set aside. Filling: Simmer dates and water together, uncovered, for five minutes. If mixture is too dry to spread easily, add a little more water. Spread carefully over bottom layer. Top layer: Beat egg whites until foamy and turning white. Add brown sugar as you continue beating until stiff. Spread over dates; sprinkle with almonds. Bake for 30 minutes. Cool; cover to store. This gives meringue time to soften. Cut with clean, sharp knife.

Nicole Cote
St. David, Maine

Applesauce Bars

"While I was an employee of USDA at the Aroostook Experimental Farm in Presque Isle, these bars were very well received by the visiting doctors from the Research Center at Beltsville, MD."

Preparation Time: 20 minutes

Baking Time: 25 to 35 minutes

32 bars

2¼   cups all-purpose flour
1   teaspoon cinnamon
¼   teaspoon ground cloves
1   teaspoon salt
2   teaspoons baking soda
1½   cups granulated sugar
½   cup butter or margarine
1½   cups applesauce
1   cup raisins
1   cup confectioners' sugar
2   tablespoons lemon juice (approximately)

Preheat oven to 375°. Sift dry ingredients together; set aside. Cream sugar and margarine until light and fluffy. Stir in applesauce. Mix well. Add sifted dry ingredients. Mix well again. Fold in raisins. Turn into well greased 9x13-inch pan. Bake for 25 to 35 minutes, or until toothpick comes out clean. After baking, mix confectioners' sugar and lemon juice and spread on bars while they are still hot.

Alice M. Dyer
Bangor, Maine

Note: These freeze well, but should not be frosted prior to freezing. Great recipe for those who must restrict their egg consumption.

Rocky Road Fudge Bars

Preparation Time: 45 minutes

Baking Time: 25 to 35 minutes

36 Bars

Bars
½   cup margarine or butter
1   ounce (1 square) unsweetened chocolate
1   cup sugar
1   cup all-purpose flour
¾   cup chopped nuts
1   teaspoon baking powder
1   teaspoon vanilla
2   eggs

Filling
6   ounces cream cheese, softened
½   cup sugar
2   tablespoons flour
¼   cup margarine or butter, softened
1   egg
½   teaspoon vanilla
⅓   cup chopped nuts
1   6-ounce package semisweet chocolate chips (optional)

Frosting
2   cups miniature marshmallows
¼   cup margarine or butter
1   ounce (1 square) unsweetened chocolate
2   ounces cream cheese, softened
¼   cup milk
3   cups powdered sugar
½   teaspoon vanilla

Preheat oven to 350°. For Bars: In large saucepan, melt margarine and chocolate over low heat. In small bowl, stir together flour and baking powder. Stir into the chocolate mixture. Add remaining bar ingredients; mix well. Spread in greased and lightly-floured 13x9-inch pan.

For Filling: In small bowl, combine all filling ingredients except nuts and chocolate chips. Beat 1 minute at medium speed until smooth and fluffy. Stir in nuts. Spread over chocolate mixture; sprinkle with chocolate chips, if desired. Bake for 25 to 30 minutes, or until toothpick comes out clean. Sprinkle with marshmallows and bake 2 minutes longer.

For Frosting: Meanwhile, in large saucepan, melt margarine, chocolate, remaining cream cheese and milk over low heat. Remove from heat. Stir in powdered sugar and vanilla until smooth. Immediately pour over marshmallows and swirl together. Chill until firm.

Judith Coffin
Millinocket, Maine

Tester's Note: This recipe is more complicated than most bars, but well worth it for special occasions. Really delicious!

Sheila's Brownies

Preparation Time: 15 minutes

Baking Time: 45 to 50 minutes

25 to 30 squares

4	ounces unsweetened chocolate
1	cup butter
2	cups sugar
3	eggs, beaten
1	teaspoon vanilla
1	cup broken walnuts
1	cup sifted flour
¼	teaspoon salt

Preheat oven to 350°. Melt chocolate and butter over hot water. Remove from heat. Add sugar, eggs and vanilla. Mix well. Stir in walnuts. Sift flour and salt. Add gradually mixing well. Pour into greased and floured 9-inch square pan. Bake for 45 to 50 minutes. Cool thoroughly before cutting into squares.

Frankie Plymale
Portland, Maine

Ginger Bars

Preparation Time: 20 minutes

Baking Time: 15 to 20 minutes

36 bars

1½ cups butter or margarine
1   cup sugar
2   eggs
½   cup molasses
2½ cups flour
½   teaspoon baking soda
2   teaspoon baking powder
½   teaspoon each ginger, cinnamon, cloves
½   cup milk
2   cups confectioners' sugar
3   tablespoons boiling water
1   teaspoon vanilla

Preheat oven to 350°. Combine butter and sugar. Add eggs and beat. Add molasses. Sift together all dry ingredients and stir into butter mixture in 3 parts, alternating with milk. Bake in greased 11x17-inch pan for 15 to 20 minutes. Mix together confectioners' sugar, water and vanilla. Frost while warm. Cool and cut into bars.

Ann Dynan
Old Greenwich, Connecticut

Note: Easy to prepare and makes lots of bars. They freeze well.

caramelitas

"For many years my husband and our seven children raced sled dogs with the New England Sled Dog Club. Caramelitas were standard fare on race weekends and now are our traditional 'comfort food'. This recipe can be halved and can also be frozen. Easier to cut when still a little warm."

Preparation Time: 30 minutes

Baking Time: 30 minutes

24 to 36 bars

2   cups plus 6 tablespoons flour, divided
2   cups quick oats
3   sticks margarine, melted
1½ cups brown sugar
1   teaspoon salt
1   12-ounce bag chocolate chips
1   cup walnuts, chopped
1   12¼-ounce jar caramel ice cream topping

Preheat oven to 350°. Mix 2 cups flour, oats, melted margarine, brown sugar and salt together. Pack half into well-greased 11x17-inch pan. Bake 10 minutes. Remove from oven. Sprinkle chocolate chips and walnuts over the top. Mix caramel topping with remaining 6 tablespoons flour and drizzle over nuts and chocolate chips. Top with remaining half of crumbs and pat down gently. Bake 20 minutes longer.

Anne Minster
Norway, Maine

Marble Squares

"When we came in from sledding, the grandchildren always went directly to Grammy's stash of homemade cookies. These marble squares proved to be the best re-energizer for the next round of sledding. Sit by a wood stove with a marble square and a glass of milk and you'll surely feel like it's winter in Maine!"

Preparation Time: 30 minutes

Baking Time: 25 to 30 minutes

24 to 32 squares

½	cup butter or margarine
¾	cup water
1½	1-ounce squares unsweetened chocolate
1	8-ounce package cream cheese, softened
2⅓	cups sugar, divided
3	eggs
2	cups flour
1	teaspoon baking soda
½	teaspoon salt
½	cup sour cream
1	6-ounce package semi-sweet chocolate chips

Preheat oven to 375°. Melt butter, water and chocolate in a large saucepan over low heat. Cool. Combine cream cheese, ⅓ cup sugar and 1 egg. Mix well. Set aside. Put flour, 2 cups of sugar, baking soda, and salt into a sifter. Sift into chocolate mixture in several batches, stirring after each addition. Beat in remaining 2 eggs and sour cream. Spread batter into a greased and floured 15½x10½-inch jelly-roll pan. Spoon the cream cheese mixture over the top. Cut through with a knife to create a marbled effect. Sprinkle chocolate bits over the top. Bake for 25 to 30 minutes.

Martha Leslie Long
Henderson, North Carolina

Brownies

"This is an old family recipe."

Preparation Time: 35 minutes

Baking Time: 25 to 25 minutes

15 to 20 large squares

1   cup melted butter
1¼ cups sugar
2   teaspoons vanilla
4   eggs
1   cup sifted flour
⅔   cup cocoa
½   teaspoon baking powder
¼   teaspoon salt
½   cup chopped nuts
1-2 16-ounce cans chocolate frosting

Preheat oven to 350°. Blend butter, sugar and vanilla in mixing bowl. Add eggs, beat well with spoon. In separate bowl combine flour, cocoa, baking powder, and salt. Gradually add dry ingredients to liquid mixture and stir until blended. Add nuts. Spread mixture into greased 9x13-inch baking dish. Bake for 20 to 25 minutes. Cool and then ice with the amount of frosting you like.

Mary Casagrande
Scarborough, Maine

One Bowl Brownies

Preparation Time: 15 minutes

Baking Time: 30 to 35 minutes

3 dozen

4	ounces unsweetened chocolate
1½	sticks margarine or butter
2	cups sugar
3	eggs
1	teaspoon vanilla
1	cup flour
1½	cups chopped pecans or walnuts

Preheat oven to 350°. Microwave chocolate and margarine in large microwavable bowl on high for 2 minutes or until margarine is melted. Stir until chocolate is completely melted. Stir sugar into chocolate until completely mixed. Mix in flour until well blended. Stir in nuts. Spread in greased 9x13-inch pan. Bake for 30 to 35 minutes, or until toothpick inserted into center comes out with fudgy crumbs. Do not overbake. Cool in pan and cut into squares.

Joan Stockford
Cape Elizabeth, Maine

Frosted Fudge Brownies

Preparation Time: 15 minutes

Baking Time: 30 minutes

¾ cup sifted flour
½ cup shortening, softened
5 tablespoons cocoa
1 teaspoon vanilla
1 cup sugar
½ teaspoon salt
2 eggs
½ cup chopped walnuts

Topping
5 tablespoons butter, softened, divided
2 cups sifted confectioners' sugar
2 tablespoons cream
1 teaspoon vanilla
1 ounce unsweetened baking chocolate

Preheat oven to 350°. Place all ingredients except nuts in large bowl of electric mixer and beat until thoroughly blended. Add nuts and allow to just blend in. Put the stiff batter into a greased 8-inch square pan and spread evenly. Bake for 30 minutes. Cool slightly. Topping: Brown 4 tablespoons butter over medium heat. Blend with confectioners' sugar. Blend in cream and vanilla. Spread over cooled brownies. Melt baking chocolate with remaining 1 tablespoon butter. When cooled spread in a very thin glaze over top of frosted brownies.

Dot Cleveland
South Portland, Maine

Butterscotch Brownies

Preparation Time: 15 minutes

Baking Time: 20 to 25 minutes

16 squares

¼ cup margarine or butter
1 cup light brown sugar
1 egg
½ cup flour
1 teaspoon baking powder
½ teaspoon salt
½ teaspoon vanilla
½ cup coarsely chopped walnuts

Preheat oven to 350°. Melt margarine over low heat; stir in brown sugar and allow to cool. Stir in egg. Sift together all dry ingredients and add to margarine and sugar mixture. Beat in thoroughly, then add vanilla and chopped nuts, stirring to distribute evenly. Spread in greased and floured 8-inch square baking pan. Bake for 20 to 25 minutes. They will appear soft. Allow to cool about 5 minutes and then cut into squares.

Dot Cleveland
South Portland, Maine

Molasses Cookies

"This was my grandmother's recipe which my own mother baked on the days when my children got off the school bus at her house. They are good at Christmas with colored sugar on them."

Preparation Time: 1 hour

Baking Time: 8 to 10 minutes per cookie sheet

6 dozen

1	cup sugar
1	cup molasses
1	teaspoon soda
1	cup cold water
1	cup shortening, melted
5½	cups sifted flour
1	teaspoon ginger
½	teaspoon salt
1	egg
	Dash lemon juice
	Sugar to sprinkle

Mix first 3 ingredients together and let sit for a minute. Mix in next 5 ingredients. Add the egg and lemon juice. Chill overnight. Preheat oven to 350°. Roll out, cut and sprinkle sugar on cookies before baking. Bake for 8 to 10 minutes.

Gloria P. Ramp
Bangor, Maine

Old Fashioned Molasses Cookies

"These cookies used to be a favorite with my Dad. He liked to have one or two with a glass of cold milk as a mid-morning snack. Mom made a batch nearly every other day when we six children were growing up. Of course, the neighbor kids helped take care of a few also."

Preparation Time: 30 minutes

Baking Time: 5 to 6 minutes per cookie sheet

5 dozen

1	cup molasses
½	cup sugar
½	cup cold water
1	egg
½	cup oil
4-5	cups flour
2	teaspoons soda
1	teaspoon cream of tartar
½	teaspoon cinnamon
¼	teaspoon ginger
¼	teaspoon salt

Preheat oven to 400°. Mix together molasses, sugar and cold water. Add egg and oil. Sift together the flour, soda, cream of tartar, cinnamon, ginger and salt, and add to the other ingredients. Divide dough in half and turn onto floured cloth to prevent sticking. Roll dough to about ¼-inch thick. Cut with cookie cutter. Bake on ungreased cookie sheet for 5 to 6 minutes.

Lola Crockett for Marion Billings
Bethel, Maine

Downeast Molasses Sugar Cookies

"This recipe was given to us by a baker, many years ago."

Preparation Time: 20 minutes

Baking Time: 8 to 10 minutes per cookie sheet

3 dozen

1	cup sugar
¼	cup molasses
1	egg
½	cup margarine
2	cups sifted flour
2	teaspoon baking soda
1	teaspoon cinnamon
1	teaspoon ginger
½	teaspoon cloves
¼	teaspoon salt
	Sugar to sprinkle

Preheat oven to 375°. Mix first four ingredients together well. Mix remaining ingredients together and then add to first mixture. Drop by teaspoonfuls on ungreased cookie sheet about 2 inches apart. Sprinkle with sugar. Bake for 8 to 10 minutes. After baking they won't look well done. Just leave them on cookie sheet for two minutes and then take them off.

Chrystel H. Buck
Poland, Maine

Stone Jar Molasses Cookies

"Made without eggs, this was a popular wartime recipe"

Preparation Time: 15 minutes

Baking Time: 5 to 8 minutes per cookie sheet

5 dozen 2½-inch cookies

1	cup molasses
½	cup lard or shortening
1	teaspoon soda
2¼	cups flour
1¾	teaspoons baking powder
1½	teaspoons ginger
1	teaspoon salt

Bring molasses to boil. Remove from heat and add lard (or shortening) and soda and blend. Sift dry ingredients into mixture. Mix well. Chill 2 to 4 hours. Preheat oven to 350°. Roll 1/16-inch thick. Cut with cookie cutter. Bake on lightly-greased cookie sheet for 5 to 8 minutes.

Gail Flaherty
Rockland, Maine

Tester's Note: Great for decorating as holiday cookies - gingerbread men, etc.

Thin Molasses Cookies

"My sister often made these cookies to serve with tea to her visitors. I find they are a favorite with my friends, too."

Preparation Time: 15 minutes

Baking Time: 7 to 8 minutes per cookie sheet

2 dozen

1	egg
1	cup white sugar
¾	cup melted shortening
4	tablespoons molasses
2	cups flour
2	teaspoons soda
1	teaspoon cinnamon
½	teaspoon ginger

Preheat oven to 325°. Mix the first four ingredients well. Sift and add remaining ingredients. Make small balls and drop on cookie pan. Press down. Bake for 7 or 8 minutes.

Kay Marstaller
Camden, Maine

Ginger Snaps

"My dad, Arnold Dyer, was an Alzheimer's patient and since his death this recipe is even more important to me. This was his favorite recipe to make for his grandkids and all his friends. He would methodically dust each and every one of them to remove every speck of flour that may have been left on the cookie after baking. For Dad presentation was everything."

Preparation Time: 30 minutes

Baking Time: 5 to 6 minutes per cookie sheet

7 to 10 dozen cookies, depending on size of cutter

1	cup molasses
½	cup sugar
1	egg
2	teaspoons soda
2	teaspoons ginger
½	teaspoon cinnamon
⅔	cup shortening
	Flour for kneading

Preheat oven to 350°. Mix first 7 ingredients. Knead in enough flour to prevent sticking. Roll very thin. Cut with your favorite cutter. Bake for 5 to 6 minutes.

Judi Collier
Bangor, Maine

Soft Spicy Hermits

"These were, by far, my husband's favorite sweet."

Preparation Time: 20 minutes

Baking Time: 20 to 25 minutes

½	cup salad oil
½	cup molasses
1	cup sugar
½	teaspoon salt
3	cups flour
¼	teaspoon cloves
1	teaspoon cinnamon
½	teaspoon nutmeg
1	teaspoon soda
½	cup milk
¾	cup raisins

Preheat oven to 350°. Beat salad oil, molasses, sugar and salt. Mix flour, spices and soda. Add to oil mixture, alternating with milk. Add raisins. This can be spread on a cookie sheet in ribbon fashion and cut for hermits, made as soft cookies or made as bar cookies. Bake for 20 to 25 minutes. Do not overbake.

Marjorie Jamback
Biddeford, Maine

Butter Sugar Cookies

"These cookies are wonderful and have been a favorite with my children over the years. Many times we have enjoyed decorating them together. They were even a requested treat for care packages during my son's college days. I now look forward to introducing them to my first grandchild, Lauren."

Preparation Time: 15 minutes

Baking Time: 10 to 12 minutes per cookie sheet

5 dozen 2½-inch cookies

½	cup real butter (room temperature)
1	cup sugar
2	eggs
1	teaspoon vanilla
3	cups all-purpose flour
½	teaspoon salt
2	teaspoons baking powder
2	tablespoons milk
	Icing or sugar to decorate (optional)

Cream butter and sugar together until light and fluffy. Add eggs, one at a time; beat well after each; stir in vanilla. Sift flour, salt and baking powder together; beat into creamed mixture, alternating with milk. Form dough into a ball and wrap in foil; chill overnight. Preheat oven to 350°. Divide dough into fourths and roll on well-floured board to ⅛-inch thick. Cut with cookie cutters. Place on greased baking sheet. Bake for 10 to 12 minutes. Ice and decorate, if desired, when completely cool. Store in the refrigerator. Cookies taste best chilled.

Karen Brown
Belfast, Maine

Sour Cream Sugar Cookies

"Dad's favorite"

Preparation Time: 15 minutes

Baking Time: 15 to 25 minutes per cookie sheet

4 dozen

1   cup sugar
½   cup butter or margarine, melted
1   egg
1   cup sour cream
     Lemon flavoring
2½ cups flour
1   teaspoon soda
1   teaspoon baking powder
½   teaspoon salt

Preheat oven to 400°. Cream sugar and butter. Add egg. Add sour cream and lemon flavoring. Mix dry ingredients together and add to sour cream mixture. Chill, if necessary. Roll quite thick and bake for 15 to 25 minutes.

Sue Littlefield
Market Square Health Care Center

Filled Cookies

Preparation time: 50 minutes

Baking Time: 10 to 12 minutes per cookie sheet

3½ dozen

1	cup shortening
1	cup brown sugar
1	cup white sugar
2	eggs
1	tablespoon vanilla
3½	cups flour
1	teaspoon salt
1	teaspoon baking soda
½	teaspoon cinnamon
½	cup sour milk, or buttermilk
	Raspberry pie filling or jam

Preheat over to 350°. Cream sugars and shortening. Add eggs and vanilla. Combine dry ingredients and add, alternating with milk. Mix well. Drop by heaping teaspoonfuls onto parchment paper or greased cookie sheet. Use back of spoon to make pocket in dough. Put ½ teaspoon of filling in pocket. Place another piece of dough over top of filling. (Filling can peek out around edges.) Bake for 10 to 12 minutes.

Sandy River Center for Health and Rehabilitation
Farmington, Maine

Orange Cookies

"This is a soft cookie. Kids love them. I have had this recipe for over 30 years. It came originally from Wisconsin."

Preparation time: 30 minutes

Baking Time: 10 minutes per cookie sheet

5 dozen

¾	cup white sugar
¾	cup brown sugar
1	cup butter
2	unbeaten eggs
1	tablespoon orange juice
1	tablespoon grated orange rind
1	teaspoon vanilla
1	cup sour cream
1	teaspoon soda
3	cups flour, sifted
1	teaspoon baking powder

Frosting

2	cups powdered sugar
3	tablespoons orange juice
1	tablespoon orange rind
2	tablespoons butter

Preheat oven to 350°. Mix sugars with butter; add unbeaten eggs, one at a time, orange juice, rind and vanilla. In separate bowl mix flour and baking powder. In small bowl mix sour cream and soda. Stir flour mixture into sugar mixture, alternating with sour cream mixture. Drop by tablespoonfuls on cookie sheet. Bake for 10 minutes, or until edges are light brown. Cool. Mix frosting ingredients and frost when cool.

Sue Winters
South Thomaston, Maine

Pineapple Coconut Cookies

Preparation Time: 20 minutes

Baking Time: 8 to 10 minutes per cookie sheet

3 dozen

½   cup shortening
½   cup butter
1½ cups sugar
1   8-ounce can crushed pineapple, juice and all
1   teaspoon soda
3½ cups flour
½   teaspoon salt
1   teaspoon vanilla
1   cup coconut

Cream shortening, butter, and sugar. Add crushed pineapple. Blend soda, flour and salt and add to butter mixture. Add vanilla. Stir in coconut. Chill two hours or overnight. Preheat oven to 400°. Drop by well-rounded teaspoonfuls onto a greased cookie sheet. Bake for 8 to 10 minutes, or until tops are lightly browned.

Thelma Leavitt
Howland, Maine

Note: Can substitute ½ cup walnuts and ½ cup coconut for the 1 cup coconut, if desired.

Scottish Oat Cakes

"My mother brought this recipe home with her from a trip to Nova Scotia where there are many people of Scottish descent, as is she. This is a big recipe, but they are delicious. They are crispiest and best when rolled quite thin."

Preparation Time: 30 minutes

Baking Time: 12 to 15 minutes per cookie sheet

4 dozen

½   teaspoon soda
½   cup boiling water
2   cups flour
1   teaspoon baking powder
1   teaspoon salt
2   cups bran flakes
2   cups quick-cooking rolled oats
1¼ cups sugar
1¼ cups shortening

Preheat oven to 350°. Add soda to boiling water and let stand until cool. Mix flour, baking powder, salt, bran flakes, oats and sugar. Cut in shortening with knives. Add water/soda mixture. Roll out very thin on floured cloth or board. Cut into shapes with pastry or pizza wheel. Bake for 12 to 15 minutes, or until golden brown.

Kay White
Portland, Maine

Note: Cakes can be baked in batches, keeping remaining dough in the refrigerator for another day.

Chocolate Oatmeal Cookies

Preparation Time: 20 Minutes

Baking Time: 12 to 15 minutes per cookie sheet

3 to 4 dozen

1	cup sugar
1	cup brown sugar
¾	cup margarine
2	eggs
2	teaspoons vanilla
2	cups flour
¼	cup unsweetened cocoa
1	teaspoon baking soda
½	teaspoon baking powder
¼	cup water
2	cups oatmeal (old-fashioned or quick-cooking)

Preheat oven to 350°. Cream together sugars and margarine.
Beat in eggs and vanilla. Combine flour, cocoa, baking soda and
baking powder. Add to egg mixture, alternating with water. Stir in
oatmeal and drop from a tablespoon onto greased cookie sheet.
Bake for 12 to 15 minutes.

Norway Rehabilitation and Living Center
Norway, Maine

Chewy Brownie Cookies

Preparation Time: 5 minutes

Baking Time: 8 to 9 minutes per cookie sheet

3 to 3½ dozen

⅔   cup shortening
1½ cups light brown sugar
1   tablespoon water
1   teaspoon vanilla
2   eggs
1½ cups flour
⅓   cup unsweetened baking cocoa
¼   teaspoon baking soda
½   teaspoon salt
     Sugar to sprinkle

Preheat oven to 350°. Beat first 5 ingredients together and then add next 4 ingredients. Drop from teaspoon 1½ inches apart onto greased cookie sheet. Press lightly, if necessary, with fork and sprinkle with sugar. Bake for 8 to 9 minutes.

Esther McPhee
Rumford, Maine

Million Dollar Cookies

Preparation Time: 20 minutes

Baking Time: 10 minutes per cookie sheet

112 cookies

5	cups oatmeal
2	cups butter
2	cups sugar
2	cups brown sugar
4	eggs
1	teaspoon vanilla
4	cups flour
1	teaspoon salt
2	teaspoons baking powder
2	teaspoons soda
1	24-ounce package chocolate chips
1	8-ounce Hershey's bar, grated
3	cups chopped nuts

Preheat oven to 375°. Measure oatmeal and blend it in a blender or food processor to a fine powder. Cream butter and both sugars. Add eggs and vanilla. Mix together flour, oatmeal, salt, baking powder and soda. Add to butter mixture. Add chocolate chips, Hershey's bar and nuts. Roll into golf-ball-sized balls and place two inches apart on ungreased cookie sheet. Bake for 10 minutes.

Raylene Richard
Roxbury, Maine

Mom's Peanut Butter Cookies

"My mother, Harriet Dow, used to make these for me and my brothers."

Preparation Time: 15 minutes

Baking Time: 10 minutes per cookie sheet

1   cup shortening or butter, melted
1   cup white sugar
1   cup brown sugar
2   eggs
1   cup peanut butter
1   teaspoon vanilla
3   cups flour
2   teaspoons soda
1   teaspoon salt

Preheat oven to 350°. Cream butter and sugars. Beat in eggs. Add peanut butter. Stir in vanilla. Combine remaining ingredients and add to peanut butter mixture. Drop by spoonfuls on a lightly-greased cookie sheet. Bake for ten minutes, or until done.

Fannie Young and Renaissance Nursing Home
Franklin, Maine and Farmington, Maine

Note: Renaissance Nursing Home sent an almost identical recipe. They use an additional cup of peanut butter and ½ to 1 cup less flour. They also shape the dough into balls and flatten on the cookie sheet with a fork. Their comments about this recipe are: "When we bake, we stir everything by hand. This recipe is definitely a good aerobics workout - created a lot of laughs as we passed the bowl around - stirring, stirring, stirring!"

Peanut Butter Cup Cookies

Preparation Time: 25 minutes

Baking Time: 8 to 9 minutes per pan

3½ dozen

½ cup butter or margarine, softened
½ cup brown sugar, packed
½ cup granulated sugar
1 egg
½ cup creamy-style peanut butter
½ teaspoon vanilla
1¼ cups all-purpose flour
¾ teaspoon baking soda
½ teaspoon salt
1 13-ounce bag miniature peanut butter cups, unwrapped
    and ready to use

Combine butter, sugars, egg, peanut butter and vanilla in mixing bowl. Beat until smooth. In separate bowl, combine flour, baking soda, and salt. Add to creamed mixture. Cover dough and chill. Preheat oven to 375°. When cold enough to handle easily, roll in small (walnut-sized) balls. Place each ball in a lined (or greased) miniature muffin tin. Bake for 8 to 9 minutes. Remove from oven and gently press 1 peanut butter cup into each cookie. Cool in pan 10 minutes. Remove from pan and place on cooling rack.

Colleen Gurney
Mexico, Maine

Tester's Note: This is a great recipe for kids to make, as well as to eat.

Cream Cheese Rugelach

*"These are an all-time favorite at our pastry shop.
They fly off the shelves."*

Preparation Time: 30 minutes or more

Baking Time: 13 to 16 minutes per cookie sheet

5 dozen

2	sticks butter, softened
6	ounces cream cheese, softened
⅓	cup sugar
3¼	cups cake flour
½	teaspoon salt

Filling

½	cup chopped walnuts
⅓	cup mini chocolate chips
½	cup granulated sugar
2	teaspoons cinnamon
½	cup apricot preserves

In a food processor, combine butter, cream cheese and sugar. Process until well blended. Add cake flour and salt. Process until dough forms a ball around blades. Wrap in plastic wrap and refrigerate until firm, one hour or overnight. Preheat oven to 350°. In a small bowl combine walnuts, mini chocolate chips, granulated sugar and cinnamon. Mix well and set aside. Divide dough into 8 pieces. On floured work surface, roll out one piece of dough into 8-inch circle. Spread about 1 tablespoon preserves over dough. Sprinkle about 2 tablespoons walnut-sugar filling on top. Using a pizza wheel or sharp knife, cut into 8 wedges. Beginning at wide end, roll toward point, forming a crescent shape. Repeat with remaining dough, jam and filling. Place point side down, one inch apart, on greased cookie sheets. Bake 13 to 16 minutes, or until golden. Remove to rack and let cool completely before serving.

Grande Pastry Shop
Portland, Maine

Tester's Note: This dough is easy to work with even without a food processor. Just mix ingredients together, with a power or hand mixer, in the same order. If dough gets stiff, mix the flour in with hands.

Jewish Cookies

Preparation Time: 20 minutes

Baking Time: 20 to 25 minutes per cookie sheet

4 dozen

2	sticks butter
2	cups flour
½	teaspoon salt
¾	cup sour cream
1	egg yolk, beaten, (save egg white)
¾	cup sugar
1	teaspoon cinnamon

Cut butter into flour and salt. Add sour cream and egg yolk. Blend well. Shape into ball. Sprinkle with flour, wrap in wax paper and chill overnight. Preheat oven to 375°. Divide dough into three parts. Roll each third into circle. Mix sugar and cinnamon; sprinkle ⅓ on each circle. Cut each circle into 16 pie wedges; roll starting with wide edge. Brush with beaten egg white. Bake on greased cookie sheet for 20 to 25 minutes.

Colleen Gurney
Mexico, Maine

Holiday Cookies

Preparation Time: 15 minutes

Baking Time: 7 minutes per cookie sheet

4 dozen

5	cups flour
2	cups powdered sugar
1	cup butter
2	cups shortening
2	eggs, beaten
4	teaspoons vanilla
	Powdered sugar to decorate

Preheat oven to 400°. Sift flour and powdered sugar; cut in butter and shortening until mixture resembles a coarse meal. Add eggs and vanilla. Flour board well to knead dough, using more flour, as needed, to roll out to about ¼-inch thick. Cut into holiday shapes. Bake for 7 minutes. When cool, sprinkle with powdered sugar. (This recipe can be frozen, but don't put powdered sugar on the cookies until after they are taken out of the freezer.)

Suellen Begley Roberts
Peaks Island, Maine

Harlequin Pinwheel Cookies

"Last Christmas was the first one without my mom. Physically she is well but her mind is in another place. She is one of the many vibrant, talented, educated, and wonderful people who suffer from what we group together and call Alzheimer's Disease. She went to a nursing home this year. The whole family misses her terribly. But as we talk and reminisce, the memories are wonderful and the lessons taught by a strong and moral woman well learned. Her love of entertaining has been passed on to her daughters and their children. The following recipe was one of her favorites."

Preparation Time: 45 minutes

Baking Time: 8 to 10 minutes per cookie sheet

3 dozen

1	cup sifted flour
¾	teaspoon salt
¼	teaspoon baking powder
½	cup brown sugar, packed
¼	cup butter, softened
1	egg yolk
½	teaspoon vanilla

Filling

1	6-ounce package chocolate bits
1	teaspoon margarine
1	cup finely-chopped nuts
⅓	cup sweetened condensed milk
1	teaspoon vanilla
¼	teaspoon salt

Preheat oven to 375°. Sift together flour, salt and baking powder. Blend together brown sugar and soft butter. Beat egg yolk and vanilla into this mixture and then add flour mixture. Roll on lightly-floured board to 9x12-inch rectangle. Filling: Melt together chocolate bits and margarine. Stir in remaining ingredients and press this filling evenly over cookie dough. Roll up, starting at the

12-inch edge. Wrap in sheet of aluminum foil. Chill until firm or freeze. Cut into ¼-inch slices. Place on cookie sheet lined with foil. Bake 8 to 10 minutes.

Carol Day
Gorham, Maine

Cherry Nut Slices

Preparation Time: ½ hour plus chill time

Baking Time: 15 minutes per cookie sheet

approximately 5 dozen

1   cup powdered sugar
1   cup margarine or butter, softened
1   teaspoon vanilla
1   egg
2   cups all-purpose flour
1½ cups candied cherries, halved
1½ cups chopped pecans

In large bowl, blend well powdered sugar, margarine, vanilla and egg. Mix together flour, cherries and pecans; stir into sugar mixture. Chill dough 1 hour or longer for easier handling. Divide dough into thirds; shape each third into a roll 1½ inches in diameter. Wrap; chill for 3 hours or longer. Preheat oven to 325°. Cut dough into ¼-inch slices; place 1 inch apart on ungreased cookie sheets. Bake for 15 minutes, or until edges are lightly browned. Remove from cookie sheets immediately after baking.

Judith Coffin
Millinocket, Maine

Fran's Cinnamon Swirl Cookies

Preparation Time: 30 minutes

Baking Time: 10 minutes per cookie sheet

3 dozen

2   cups sugar
2   eggs
1   cup butter or margarine, melted
1   cup milk
3   teaspoons cream of tartar
2   teaspoons baking soda
1   teaspoon salt
1   teaspoon vanilla
1   teaspoon nutmeg
1   teaspoon grated lemon rind
4-6 cups flour
    Cinnamon and sugar mixture

Preheat oven to 350°. Combine sugar, eggs and butter in mixing bowl. Combine milk, cream of tartar and baking soda; add to butter mixture. Add salt, vanilla, nutmeg and lemon. Add flour. Roll out the dough, adding flour as needed to handle well. Sprinkle dough with cinnamon and sugar mixture; then roll up and slice to ¾-inch thickness.

Fran Clukey
Houlton, Maine

Sonhos (Dreams)

"This is an old family recipe - a Portuguese sweet served on festive occasions. They are called dreams because they fry up into funny shapes - like cloud formations."

Preparation Time: 30 minutes

3 dozen

1	cup water
1	stick unsalted butter
4	teaspoons sugar
	Dash of salt
1	cup sifted flour
4	large eggs
	Vegetable oil for deep frying
½	cup sugar
1	teaspoon cinnamon

Bring water, butter and sugar to a boil. Add flour all at once. Cook and beat with wooden spoon until mixture forms a ball. Add eggs, one at a time, beating vigorously, until mixture is smooth and shiny. Drop by teaspoonfuls into hot vegetable oil and fry until golden. Turn puff, if necessary. Drain on paper towel. Mix sugar and cinnamon. Place Sonhos in fancy dish and sprinkle with cinnamon sugar mixture.

Alvira Lagomarsino
Cape Elizabeth, Maine

Cream Puffs

"At our rehabilitation and living center we have these as a special treat after some of our games, sometimes as a prize or consolation prize where everybody wins. The residents love them."

Preparation Time: 30 minutes

Baking Time: 30 to 35 minutes

12 cream puffs

1	cup water
½	cup butter
⅛	teaspoon salt
1	cup all-purpose flour
4	eggs
	Whipped cream, pudding, or ice cream
	Powdered sugar (optional)

Preheat oven to 400°. In medium saucepan combine water, butter and salt. Bring to a boil. Add flour all at once, stirring vigorously. Cook and stir until mixture forms a ball. Remove from heat. Cool for 10 minutes. Add eggs, one at a time, beating well with a wooden spoon after each addition. Drop dough by 12 heaping tablespoons onto greased baking sheet. Bake 30 to 35 minutes, or until golden brown. Cool on wire rack. Cut tops from puffs; remove soft dough from inside. Fill with whipped cream, pudding or ice cream and replace tops. If desired, sift powdered sugar over tops.

Lynne Whitney
Norway, Maine

Tester's Note: We liked them as a dessert and, the next morning, filled the left-overs with scrambled eggs as a breakfast treat!

Meringue Kisses

"A family favorite. Great for anyone on a gluten-free diet."

Preparation Time: 10 minutes

Baking Time: 45 minutes plus several hours cooling time

2½ to 3 dozen

2   egg whites
½   cup sugar
½   teaspoon vanilla

Preheat oven to 250°. Beat egg whites until stiff; add sugar,
a little at a time, while continuing to beat. Gently fold in vanilla.
Cover cookie sheet with brown paper. (I use inside of clean paper
bag.) Drop by teaspoonfuls on brown paper. Put in oven for
45 minutes. Then turn off oven, without opening door, and leave
door closed overnight or until cold.

Annie Williamson
Yarmouth, Maine

Peanut Butter Candy Bars

Preparation Time: 1 hour

20 bars

2   sticks margarine
1   16-ounce jar peanut butter
1   pound powdered sugar
1   cup crushed graham crackers
1   12-ounce package semi-sweet chocolate chips

Melt 1 stick margarine. By hand, blend in peanut butter,
powdered sugar and graham crackers. Mixture is very thick,
Mix well and press into 9x13-inch pan. Melt remaining 1 stick
margarine; stir in chocolate chips. Pour over peanut butter
mixture and smooth. Chill, cut into small bars and enjoy!

Patricia Gardner
Peaks Island, Maine

Date Balls

"The highlight of the Christmas holidays, for my children when they were small, was Aunt Bertha's date balls. Even though my children are now married and away and Aunt Bertha has died, I still make them every year. It keeps this very dear lady with us through her special treat."

Preparation Time: 30 minutes

3 dozen

1	stick margarine, melted
1	cup chopped dates
1	cup sugar
2	eggs, beaten
3	cups Rice Krispies
1	teaspoon vanilla
	Shredded coconut
	Chopped nuts (optional)

Mix margarine, dates, sugar and eggs in a large iron fry pan. Stir constantly, cooking over low heat, for 10 minutes. Let cool for about 5 minutes. Add Rice Krispies and vanilla; mix well. Let cool 5 minutes. Shape into balls and roll in coconut and/or chopped nuts. Put cookies on tray and put in a cool place so they will firm up. Hint: Rub hands with margarine for easier handling of mixture.

Peggy Grant
Saco, Maine

Uncle Charles' Texas Chocolate Fudge

Preparation Time: 45 minutes

36 to 48 pieces

1   7½-ounce jar marshmallow fluff
1   8-ounce Hershey's milk chocolate bar, broken into pieces
1   12-ounce package semisweet chocolate chips
1-2 cups chopped nuts (pecans or walnuts) (optional)
2   teaspoons vanilla
4½ cups sugar
1   12-ounce can evaporated milk
1   stick butter
     Dash of salt

Place the marshmallow fluff, chocolate bar(s), chocolate chips, vanilla and nuts in a large bowl ready to add to the cooked ingredients. In large saucepan combine sugar, milk, butter and salt. Mix well. Place over medium heat, stirring constantly so sugar will dissolve and won't burn onto pan. Bring to rolling boil (a boil that can't be stirred down). Boil for 12 minutes, stirring constantly. Remove from heat and pour liquid over ingredients in bowl. Stir until chocolate is melted and is mixed well. Pour into a buttered 9x13-inch pan. Let cool. It hardens as it cools. This is best if it sits for a couple of days before removing from the pan.

Judith Coffin
Millinocket, Maine

Lauren's Candies

"This recipe was originally called Trudy's Candies, *but each time my daughter and I made it, she assumed it was her grandmother Gertrude's recipe. Grandma, who was diagnosed with Alzheimer's, insists that it isn't her recipe. Finally, after making this recipe every holiday season for ten years, my daughter Lauren said 'Okay, from now on we're calling them Lauren's Candies'."*

Preparation Time: 15 minutes

3 dozen cookies

1	6-ounce package chocolate chips
¼	cup peanut butter
⅓	cup coconut
½	cup chopped nuts

Heat chocolate chips in double boiler. Stir in peanut butter. Add other ingredients. Drop by teaspoonfuls onto platter lined with wax paper. Refrigerate until firm.

Barbara Berv
Denver, Colorado

Tester's Note: Great! I used natural peanut butter, which worked well. For the nuts, I used unsalted peanuts and salted cashews... it was yummy.

Toffee

"This is made every Christmas for family and friends. I make them with the Smith College Pecans and they are always a rave!"

Preparation Time: 15 minutes

2 to 3 dozen

1   cup nuts, chopped (pecans, walnuts, or almonds), divided
½   pound margarine or butter
1   cup white sugar
⅓   cup brown sugar
2   tablespoons water
¼   teaspoon soda
1½ cups chocolate bits

Butter rimmed 9x13-inch cookie sheet. Spread with ¾ cup broken nuts. In heavy saucepan melt margarine (or butter); add sugars along with water. Stir constantly until 300° on candy thermometer. Put soda in quickly and pour into pan spreading evenly. Let sit about 5 minutes. Sprinkle chocolate bits over this. When softened, spread with knife. Sprinkle remaining nuts on top. Set in refrigerator to harden. Break into any size pieces you desire. Store in tight container.

Helen Woodbrey
Gorham, Maine

Pecans

"After selling thousands of pounds of pecans for scholarships, this recipe is one of the most popular."

Preparation Time: 10 minutes

Baking Time: 1 hour

1 pound

1   egg white
1   teaspoon water
1   pound pecans
½   cup sugar
¼   teaspoon salt
½   teaspoon cinnamon

Preheat oven to 225°. In a large bowl beat egg white until frothy. Add water and beat until well mixed. Add pecans to mixture. Combine sugar, salt and cinnamon and add pecans to coat. Butter a 10x15-inch pan. Spread nuts evenly. Bake for 1 hour, stirring every 15 minutes. Stir and chill.

Janet Richardson
Portland, Maine

Popcorn Balls

*"This was my mother's 'special' every Christmas Eve.
She would wrap each ball in wax paper and place in a large
bowl on the table with love! Alzheimer's has taken her talent,
but our memories still remain!"*

Preparation Time: 30 to 45 minutes

15 to 20 popcorn balls

½	cup brown sugar
1	cup molasses
2	tablespoons vinegar
2	tablespoons margarine
½	cup cold water
¼	teaspoon baking soda
5	cups (approximately) of freshly popped unsalted popcorn

In saucepan mix sugar, molasses, vinegar, margarine and water.
Boil gently, without stirring, until a portion tested in cold water
forms a soft ball. Add soda and mix. While foamy, pour over the
popcorn. Mix thoroughly. Press together into balls about 3 inches
in diameter. Rub a piece of margarine on your hand so the corn
will not stick to you. Be careful, as mixture will be hot. Work
quickly when the candy mixture is ready. Have fun! A real treat.

Miriam Small
Venice, Florida

Tester's Note: Fun. Good to do with children and grandchildren.

Contributors

Cheri Alexander
Eleanor Allen
The Honorable Thomas Allen
Dorothy Almog
Thelma Andrews
Susan Arnold
Annette Austin
Deanne Bailey
The Honorable John Baldacci
Elizabeth Barnaby
Betsy Barrett
Shirley Bastien
Connie Batson
Jean Baxter
Katherine Beach
Andy Beauchesne
Elizabeth P. Beaulieu
Louise T. Berry
Barbara Berv
Vera Berv
BiBo's Madd Apple Café
Joanne Bingham
Rev. Judith Blanchard
Bella Blier
Nancy Bloch
Beverly Boardman
Evelyn Bodemer
Ann Bonney
Edwina S. Bonney
Lesa Borg
Boston Harbor Hotel (Chef Daniel Bruce)

Barbara Boucher
Marion Bourgoin
Ardith Bradshaw
Larry Braziel
Susan Braziel
Karen Brown
Donna Brunstad
Chrystel H. Buck
Georgina Burt
Karen Byram
Reno Byram
Melissa Canwell
Judy Carter
Casa Napoli Ristorante
Mary Casagrande
Hattie Cavanaugh
Nola Chaisson
Catherine Churchill
Churchill Caterers
Elinor Clark
Hilary Clark
Lucille Clark
Dot Cleveland
Fran Clukey
Judith Coffin
Judi Collier
The Honorable Susan Collins
Roberta Conerette
Dorothy L. Connolly
The Cornish Inn (Paul Miller, Chef)
Shirley Corse
Nicole Cote

Dorothy Crandell
Kathy Crispin
Lola Crockett
Pat Cunningham
Harriet Currie
Barbara Curtis
Marie Curtis
Gloria C. Daigle
Violet Dattner
Carolyn Davis
Carol Day
Sarah deDoes
Nan Delaney
Susu DePaolo
Joyce Dexter
Deborah Dillon
Joan Dinsmore
Cindy Dodge
Dee Dole
Suzanne Dolloff
Lyn Donahue
Jim Donahue
Sheila Donaldson
Brian M. Dorsk
Hillary Dorsk
Elizabeth Douglass
Doris Brown Dow
Kathy Dow
Gail Dransfield
Marlene Duncan
Alice Dyer
Ann Dynan
Sandy Enck

Contributors

Edith Farnum

Inez M. Farrell

Charlene Ferguson

Sally Ferko

Jan LeMessurier Flack

Gail Flaherty

Eileen Flanagan

Fore St. (Esau A. Crosby, II. Sous Chef)

Mary Lee Fowler

Marjorie Fuller

Peg Furey

Carol Furlong

Gabriel's (Gabriel Bremer)

Connie Gagne

John Gale, M.D.

Patricia Gardner

Gail Gilmore

Eleanor Goldberg

Irma Goldberg

Peggy Greenhut Golden

Lynn Goldfarb

Gloria Gove

Grande Pastry Shop

Susan Grondin

Lori S. Grant

Peggy Grant

Joni Hanson

Jane Hards

Harraseeket Inn

Virginia G. Harvey

Elizabeth Hatcher

Mary Hillas

Betsy Hillman

Rebecca Hotelling

Catherine B. Houts

Hugo's Portland Bistro (David H. Smith, Executive Chef)

Joan Hyde

The Island Inn (Chef: Duane Judson)

Marjorie Jamback

Marla Jandreau

Erma Johnson

Fran Johnson

Linda Johnson

Hazel Jolotta

Bambi Jones

Audrey Joy

Judy Kane

Marcia Kay

Joyce Kidney

Phyllis Kindt

Alan King

Ann Kirner

Connie Korda

Lake House (Michael Meyer, Innkeeper)

Pat Lambrew

Dawn Leavitt

Glenna Leavitt

Patsy Leavitt

Thelma Leavitt

Kathleen Leslie

John Leslie

Sheila Levine

Fran Lewandowski

Sue Littlefield

Nancy Lombardelli

Martha Leslie Long

Anna M. Lujan

Catherine Maas

Melody MacDonald

J. MacDonald

Patricia Maas Major

Donna Marchinetti

Market Square Health Care Center

Kay Marstaller

Krista Martin

Constance McCabe

Carolyn Cooper McGoldrick

Elizabeth McLeod

Denise McLeod

Ester McPhee

Tonia Nadzo Medd

Anne Minster

Christine M. Munsey

Reajean Murphy

Barbara Nelson

Susan Nielson

Patricia Noonan

Norway Rehabilitation and Living Center

Ann Noyes

Donna Oakes

Stella Ouellette

Marilyn Paige

Genevieve Palmer

Contributors

Darla Patheaude
Barbara Payson
Christy Peters
Janet Philbrick
Polly Pierce
Lisa Plotkin
Frankie Plymale
Penny Porter
Barbara Pratt
Harriet H. Price
Shirley Quinlan
Carol Rabinovitz
Gloria P. Ramp
Anita Reardon
Ada Recknagel
Carol Reidy
Renaissance Nursing Home
Gerri Reny
Grace Reny
Raylene Richard
Janet Richardson
Helen Riddle
Sybil Riemensnider
Suellen Begley Roberts
Carol Rodgers
Charlotte Rose
Rose Buse Ross
Hilde H. Royer
Donna Rubin
Althea Sage
Sandy River Center for Health & Rehabilitaion
Virginia Scheckel

Barbara Schenkel
Joan Dow Scott
Phyllis Scribner
Virginia M. Self
Sally Sewall
Veronica Sheehan
Elaine Fantle Shimberg
Brenda Sickles
Joe Sirois
Betty A. Small
Miriam Small
Elaine Smith
Erna Smith
Debra Soubble
Lorraine Soucy
Alice Spencer
Hope Stacey
Ruby Stambaugh
Joan Stockford
Stone Soup (Chefs: Chris Cole & Caite Maynard)
Stonewall Kitchen
Sally Subilia
Sudbury Inn (Cheri Thurston)
Mary Taddia
Tall Pines Rehabilitation & Living Center
Debby Taylor
Marilyn Tenney
Barbara Thelin
The Therrien Children
Bibi Thompson

Dr. Philip Thompson
Peggy Thompson
Connie Thurston
Diane Tinkham
Evelyn Towne
Constance Turcotte
Sheryl Varsanen
Priscilla Verrier
Jean Vetter
Elinor Vigue
Mary Anne Vitalius
Barb Viti
Diane Voisine
Diane Volk
Kathy Walsh
Kathy Warman
The Waterford Inne (Barbara Vanderzanden)
Liz Weaver
Joy & Crystal Welch
Carol Jamback Weldin
Tish Whipple
Kay White
Lynne Whitney
Margaret Wilkis
Annie Williamson
Sue Winters
Helen Woodbrey
Christine Wright
Polly Wright
Jill Wyman
Fannie Young

Index

O

P

R

RAISINS

RASPBERRIES

RHUBARB

RICE

S

SALADS

SALMON

MAINE ALZHEIMER'S ASSOCIATION
COOKBOOK ORDER FORM

Mail To: Maine Alzheimer's Association
163 Lancaster Street, Suite 160B
Portland, Maine 04101
Please send me *"I Remember..."*, the Maine Alzheimer's Association Cookbook:
(Available Fall, 1999)

Ship To (If different address):

Name _____   Name _____

Address _____   Address _____

_____   _____

Telephone _____

Payment must accompany order.
Make checks payable to: Maine Alzheimer's Association.
All credit card orders must be confirmed by faxing a completed copy of this order form to:
Maine Alzheimer's Association—207-772-0354
Please charge my MasterCard or Visa *(Circle One)*

	Qty	Price	Total
Cardholder Name _____	_____	$18.95/Ea.	_____
Account No. _____		Shipping and Handling (from chart below) _____	
Expiration Date _____		Maine residents add 5.5% sales tax @ $1.05 per book _____	
Authorized Signature _____		Total Amount Enclosed _____	

* *

Shipping and Handling Chart:

Book Quantity	Within New England	Outside New England
1–3	4.00	7.00
4–6	8.00	11.00
7–9	12.00	15.00
each additional 3	(add) 4.00	(add) 7.00

* *